Understanding

# Arthritis
# and Rheumatism

Doctor Jennifer G. Worrall

Publish
in asso

**IMPORTANT**
This book is intended not as a substitute for personal
medical advice but as a supplement to that advice for
the patient who wishes to understand more about his
or her condition.

Before taking any form of treatment
YOU SHOULD ALWAYS CONSULT YOUR MEDICAL
PRACTITIONER.

In particular (without limit) you should note that
advances in medical science occur rapidly and some
information about drugs and treatment contained in this
booklet may very soon be out of date.

© Family Doctor Publications 2001–2008
Updated 2002, 2003, 2005, 2006, 2008

Family Doctor Publications, PO Box 4664, Poole, Dorset BH15 1NN

**ISBN-13: 978 1 903474 29 7**
**ISBN-10: 1 903474 29 9**

# Contents

Introduction ............................................... 1

Getting a diagnosis ...................................... 8

Osteoarthritis ............................................ 15

Rheumatoid arthritis .................................. 21

Gout ......................................................... 30

Other forms of inflammatory arthritis ........... 36

Other inflammatory conditions ..................... 41

Non-inflammatory conditions ....................... 45

Treating arthritis and rheumatism ................ 71

Living with arthritis and rheumatism ............ 94

Useful information .................................... 112

Index ..................................................... 126

Your pages .............................................. 139

# About the author

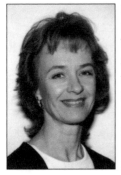

**Doctor Jennifer G. Worrall** is Consultant Rheumatologist at Whittington Hospital NHS Trust and Honorary Senior Lecturer at the Royal Free and University College Medical School, London. Her work covers all aspects of general rheumatology. Other interests are clinical effectiveness and scientific methodology.

# Introduction

## The locomotor system

The bones, joints and muscles of the body make up the locomotor system, which enables us to move around. All sorts of problems may develop in this system, particularly as we get older. Although only 3 per cent of people under 60 years of age have joint pain or stiffness, the figure rises to almost 50 per cent of people aged over 75.

## What is arthritis and rheumatism?

'Arthritis' refers to problems with the joints. There are many forms of arthritis, ranging from mild to serious, and not all of them get progressively worse. 'Rheumatism' is a vaguer term with no precise medical meaning, which refers generally to aches and pains and problems with the soft tissues, such as muscles and tendons, rather than with the joints.

   The aim of this book is to help you understand how your locomotor system works, what can go wrong with it and what help is available if it does. I hope especially to show you that there is a lot that you can

# The human skeleton

The human skeleton is able to move so well because it has many joints. These tend to degenerate over time and can cause pain and discomfort.

**BONES**

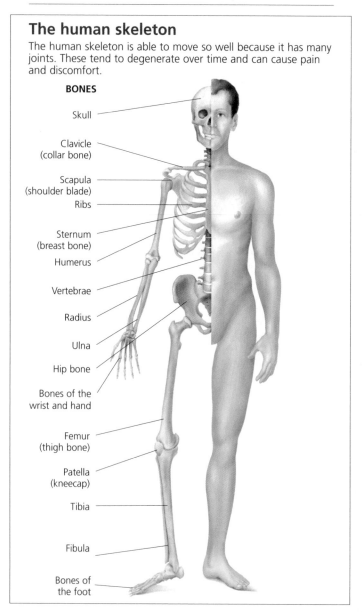

- Skull
- Clavicle (collar bone)
- Scapula (shoulder blade)
- Ribs
- Sternum (breast bone)
- Humerus
- Vertebrae
- Radius
- Ulna
- Hip bone
- Bones of the wrist and hand
- Femur (thigh bone)
- Patella (kneecap)
- Tibia
- Fibula
- Bones of the foot

do to help yourself, both to treat problems when they arise and to prevent them.

The problems of arthritis and rheumatism are not confined to older people – many common conditions affect people of all ages. Even people who do not have problems can learn to look after their joints better and so avoid problems in the future. So I hope that you will find something of interest to you whatever your age and whether or not you have arthritis. On page 112, you will find a list of addresses for further information.

## How your joints work
### Synovial joints

Joints hold the bones together and generally allow movement. Some joints, such as those in the pelvis, do not move very much and those in your skull do not move at all. But many joints can move freely and those that do are called 'synovial joints'. All of the most important joints in the body are of this type and have the same basic structure (see below). They are capable of a wide range of movement and come in many different shapes and sizes – compare the joints in your finger with those in your knees, for example; the joints look different but are made up of the same basic elements.

The ends of the two bones forming the joint are covered by cartilage. This is a gristly material which acts as a shock absorber and helps the bones to move smoothly over each other. The bones are held together by very strong ligaments and the whole joint is contained in a bag called a 'capsule'. The inside of the capsule is covered with a lining called 'synovium' (hence the name 'synovial joint') which forms a slippery surface and so allows the joint to move easily. The joint capsule contains a small amount of

## Synovial joints

Although the synovial joints in your body come in a wide range of shapes and sizes, they are nevertheless made up of the same basic elements.

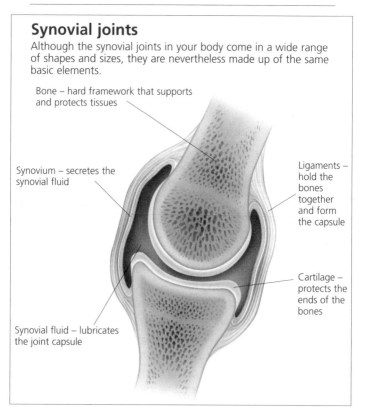

Bone – hard framework that supports and protects tissues

Synovium – secretes the synovial fluid

Synovial fluid – lubricates the joint capsule

Ligaments – hold the bones together and form the capsule

Cartilage – protects the ends of the bones

lubricating liquid, called 'synovial fluid', which is produced by the synovium.

When a joint moves, the muscles and tendons around it need to slide easily over each other and this smooth action is helped by structures called 'bursas'. A bursa is a flattened sac, rather like a balloon before it has been blown up. It contains a small amount of synovial fluid, which makes the internal surfaces slippery and allows them to slide over each other. Many tendons run in lubricated sheaths, also lined by synovium (see diagram on page 6).

## Smooth joint movement: bursas and synovial fluid

Left knee, seen from the left side. Bursas are flattened sacs, containing synovial fluid which makes them slippery, allowing the muscles and tendons to slide easily over each other when the joint moves.

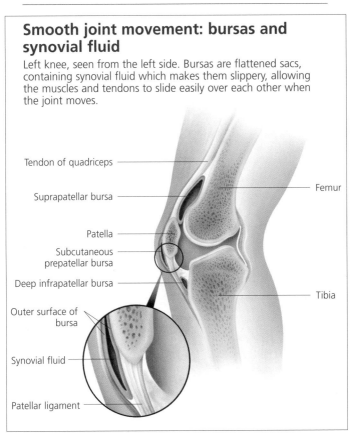

Tendon of quadriceps

Suprapatellar bursa

Femur

Patella

Subcutaneous prepatellar bursa

Deep infrapatellar bursa

Tibia

Outer surface of bursa

Synovial fluid

Patellar ligament

## Case history: Alan

Alan went to his GP because he started feeling a pain in his groin whenever he walked any distance, and thought he might have developed a hernia. After examining him, Alan's doctor found that his right hip was rather stiff and sent him for an X-ray. This showed that, at 70, Alan had mild osteoarthritis in his right hip joint. His GP advised him to take simple pain-killers when necessary but stressed the importance of

## Tendons

Many tendons run in lubricated sheaths, also lined by synovium, and lubricated by synovial fluid. The sheaths of the underside of the right hand are shown in blue.

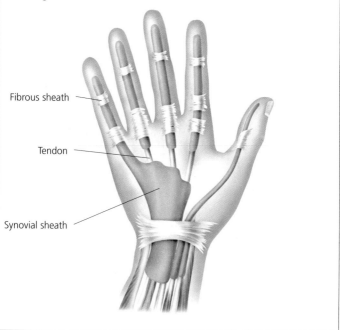

Fibrous sheath

Tendon

Synovial sheath

keeping active and taking regular exercise. Alan joined an over-50s swimming group at his local leisure centre and, after a few weeks of regular sessions, he found the groin pain much less troublesome.

## Case history: Cathy

Cathy was just 35 when she noticed that her hands were becoming swollen and painful. She also felt tired and under the weather and very stiff all over her body first thing in the morning. After about six weeks, it was taking her an hour and a half to get going in the morning, and this was a problem as she needed to get her children off to school. She saw her GP and eventually investigations revealed that she had rheumatoid arthritis. Cathy was referred to hospital where the consultant started her on drugs to ease the pain and swelling and to slow the progress of her condition. Cathy saw a physiotherapist, who advised her on suitable exercise to keep her joints working, and she saw an occupational therapist, who advised her on ways of doing her daily tasks to limit the strain on her joints. She had to attend the outpatient clinic regularly for monitoring and, after a few weeks, her symptoms were far less of a problem than before.

## KEY POINTS

- Arthritis is very common and there are many different types

- There is a lot of help – including self-help – available for arthritis sufferers

- All joints that move freely have the same basic structure

- The soft tissues making up a joint – ligaments, cartilage, capsule and the lining of the joint or synovium – are just as important as the bones

# Getting a diagnosis

## What are the symptoms?

When your locomotor system goes wrong, you feel pain and stiffness and you may notice swelling of your joints. Symptoms can be very troublesome, even disabling, and can sometimes be out of all proportion to the seriousness of the condition.

Pain, in particular, is a complex symptom and can be made much worse by stress, anxiety or depression. It is important to recognise these influences and not just assume that your arthritis must be getting worse.

Expectations can also play a part here. If you had watched an older relative gradually become disabled by painful arthritis, perhaps in the days before we had effective treatments, then, at the first sign of the inevitable aches and pains of middle age, you might become worried and upset that the same fate awaits you. Your anxiety and distress would make your pain much worse, and pain is by far the most disabling symptom – joints that are structurally sound may be almost useless if every movement causes severe pain. Fortunately, we now understand a great deal about joint symptoms and arthritis, and we have lots of treatments and advice to help sufferers lead normal lives.

When you go to your doctor with pain, stiffness or swelling of a joint, your doctor will need quite a lot of information from you and may order various tests to establish the cause of the problem. Pain in or around a joint (known medically as 'arthralgia') doesn't necessarily mean that you have arthritis. Other diseases can produce this kind of symptom. Flu, for example, can cause severe aching pain in the joints and muscles but the pain disappears as you recover.

## Seeing the doctor
### Taking your history
When you first talk to a doctor about your problems, he or she will check your symptoms and your past record of health. This is called 'taking your history'.

Your doctor will also want to know whether any close relatives have arthritis. Your family history is relevant because some people inherit a genetic susceptibility to some forms of arthritis. You should also tell your doctor if you have had any past injury to the joint, because this may cause problems to develop later on.

Certain other conditions may be associated with the onset of arthritis, such as the skin disease psoriasis or the bowel condition ulcerative colitis. Sometimes, arthritis can follow an infection – when it is called 'reactive arthritis' – so it is important to mention any recent foreign travel in case you may have picked up an infection that could account for your symptoms.

Try to be as exact as you can when describing your symptoms – when they began, whether anything triggered them, whether they are constant or intermittent, whether anything makes them better or worse, what treatment you have tried so far and what effect it had, including side effects.

## Physical examination

Your doctor may need to examine you thoroughly, even if you have only a single painful joint, because other joints may be similarly affected, even if they are not painful at the moment. Sometimes, a problem in one joint can cause strain in nearby joints.

Although these joints are normal, they become painful. For example, shoulder pain may be caused by a problem in the neck, back pain can arise from knee or hip problems, which are affecting the way you walk, and your knee may hurt even though the real problem is actually in your hip joint.

During the examination, your doctor will be looking for swelling, tenderness, stiffness of the joint and whether the joint is stable, which involves checking the muscles and ligaments that hold the joint in position. Your doctor may also take the opportunity to do other routine checks, such as measuring your blood pressure.

## Tests and investigations

Very often, your doctor will be able to identify your problem without the need for any tests, especially if only one joint is painful or if the diagnosis is obvious and straightforward. Otherwise, the tests that you have will depend on individual circumstances, but may include some or all of the following.

## Blood tests
### Full blood count
A machine counts the number of red and white blood cells and platelets in a cubic millimetre of blood.

## Taking a blood test

A blood test can provide your doctor with a great deal of information to assist with diagnosis.

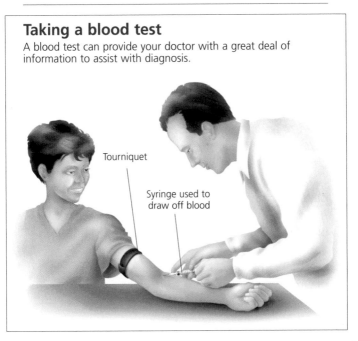

Tourniquet

Syringe used to draw off blood

The haemoglobin level in the red blood cells is also measured. This shows whether you are anaemic, as can happen in rheumatoid arthritis. Anaemia is a disorder in which haemoglobin (the oxygen-carrying component of red blood cells) is deficient or abnormal. A full blood count also measures the number of white cells in the blood, which can be increased in infection.

### Erythrocyte sedimentation rate (ESR)

Blood consists of cells and fluid (plasma). The most numerous blood cells are red blood cells which transport oxygen round the body. The ESR measures the stickiness of the red blood cells. A raised ESR suggests that inflammation is present, although it gives no indication as to the cause. The ESR is raised in those types of arthritis where the joints are severely inflamed. In osteoarthritis, which is the most common form of arthritis, inflammation is absent or mild and so the ESR is normal.

## Uric acid

This is the substance that forms crystals in the joints during attacks of gout. The level of uric acid in the blood is often raised in gout sufferers.

## Rheumatoid factor

Rheumatoid factor is an antibody that appears in the blood in some people with rheumatoid arthritis. It can also be found in low levels in normal people, especially as they get older, and in some relatives of people with rheumatoid arthritis. Rheumatoid factor does not cause disease but it can be a useful marker.

## X-rays

X-rays are not always needed to make a diagnosis of arthritis. Most people over the age of 50 have some degree of osteoarthritis and joint pain is not always related to changes seen on the X-ray.

Most forms of arthritis begin by affecting the soft tissues of the joint, such as the cartilage in osteoarthritis and the synovium in rheumatoid arthritis. Soft tissues are not easily seen on an X-ray. The X-ray is of most use in showing whether the arthritis has progressed to affect the bones and as a baseline against which future changes can be measured.

The X-ray of a joint with arthritis may show the following changes.

# X-ray investigation

An X-ray is of the most use in showing whether the arthritis has progressed to affect the bones; it also provides a baseline against which future changes can be measured.

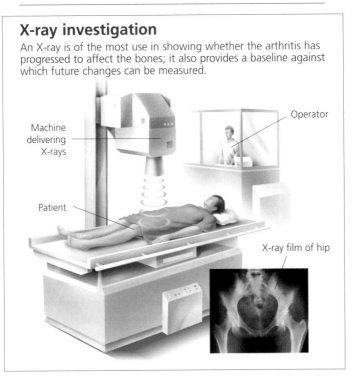

Machine delivering X-rays

Operator

Patient

X-ray film of hip

### Reduced joint space

The space between the bones of the joint is normally filled with cartilage, which cannot be seen on an X-ray. In many forms of arthritis, but especially in osteoarthritis, the cartilage becomes thinner and the joint space becomes narrower.

### Erosions

These are holes in the bones of the joint and they occur in advanced arthritis. Erosions can occur in rheumatoid arthritis and other forms of arthritis where the joints are severely inflamed. They are very unusual in osteoarthritis.

## Bony overgrowth (osteophytes)

Sometimes, arthritis causes extra bone to grow at the edges of affected joints. This can be seen quite clearly on an X-ray. In the spine, the extra bone can cause pinching of a nerve, leading to pain along the route of the nerve.

## Putting it all together

A careful history and examination, together with a few simple tests, are often all that your GP needs to make a diagnosis. Sometimes this is not possible and you will need to see a hospital specialist. However, even the specialist may not be able to make a diagnosis on the first consultation and the full picture becomes clear only with the passage of time. You will be given treatment to ease your pain and stiffness – and a period of observation, perhaps with a repeat of some of the tests, can help to establish a diagnosis.

The specialist whom you see may be a rheumatologist who specialises in inflammatory disease and the medical treatment of arthritis and rheumatism. Or he or she may be an orthopaedic surgeon if your problems are the result of injury or mechanical damage rather than inflammatory disease.

## KEY POINTS

- A careful history and examination help your doctor to make a diagnosis

- Blood tests and X-rays may help but they are not always needed

# Osteoarthritis

## How common is osteoarthritis?

Osteoarthritis is very common and affects most of us as we get older. It is the most common form of arthritis in people over the age of 65. Men are more likely to be affected than women before they reach 45, but, in the over-55s, the balance shifts so that more women are affected.

Osteoarthritis is sometimes called 'wear-and-tear arthritis' and 'degenerative arthritis', but wear and tear and degeneration are not the whole story. Lots of people who have done heavy work all their lives do not develop osteoarthritis and it is not confined to older people.

## Does it run in families?

Osteoarthritis can run in families and, if your parents had it, you have a slightly greater chance of developing it too. It can also develop early in any joint that has previously been seriously injured. Footballers, for instance, often suffer repeated cartilage injuries and may develop osteoarthritis in their knees. Besides the knee, osteoarthritis is common in the hip, the knuckle joint of the big toe, the joint at the base of the thumb, the spine, especially the lower back, and the neck.

## What's going on?

Osteoarthritis was once seen as a natural and inevitable consequence of ageing, but we now know that the real picture is rather more complex. Doctors now think that osteoarthritis may be a disorder affecting the cells responsible for making cartilage. The cartilage loses its slippery surface, cracks develop and it becomes roughened (see diagram opposite).

Over time, the cartilage becomes thinner and the joint may not move as freely as it did. The bone at the edges of the joint may change shape and bony lumps, or osteophytes, may form. In advanced cases, the cartilage may disappear entirely and the bones forming the joint may become deformed.

Women who have a family history of the condition are likely to develop problems in the joints of their fingers and thumbs and in their knees. In some people, joint problems are more widespread, with hands, feet, hips, knees and shoulders all being affected. Sometimes, a single joint such as the knee may be the only one affected, especially if it has been previously injured.

## Symptoms

Many people have no symptoms at all and find out that they have osteoarthritis only when an X-ray is taken for some other reason. Most people, however, do have some symptoms (see page 18).

Despite their knobbly appearance and the stiffness and pain, arthritic joints can continue to give good

# Osteoarthritis – what is going on?

Osteoarthritis is often referred to as wear and tear of the joints.

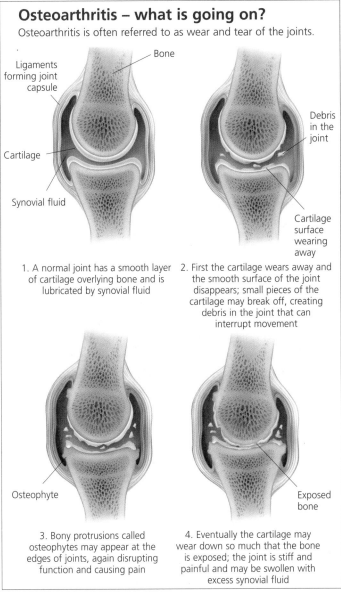

1. A normal joint has a smooth layer of cartilage overlying bone and is lubricated by synovial fluid

2. First the cartilage wears away and the smooth surface of the joint disappears; small pieces of the cartilage may break off, creating debris in the joint that can interrupt movement

3. Bony protrusions called osteophytes may appear at the edges of joints, again disrupting function and causing pain

4. Eventually the cartilage may wear down so much that the bone is exposed; the joint is stiff and painful and may be swollen with excess synovial fluid

## Common symptoms in osteoarthritis

- The joint is painful after exercise and at the end of the day, but the pain gets better with rest.
- The joint is stiff first thing in the morning or after a daytime rest, but quickly loosens up with exercise.
- The joint creaks or grinds when you move it – this is known as 'crepitus'. Crepitus is often not painful and should not prevent you from using the joint.
- Tender lumps may appear on the small joints at the ends of your fingers and the bases of your thumbs.

service for many years. Occasionally these joints, especially the knees, may suddenly become swollen and very painful, especially after some vigorous activity, such as a day out walking. The inflammation is usually mild and should respond to an anti-inflammatory drug and a short period of rest. Sometimes, the excess fluid in the joint needs to be removed and an injection of steroid given to settle the inflammation.

Arthritis in the neck may cause irritation of a nerve root, leading to numbness, pins and needles and pain in the arms. Headaches can also occur and are the result of tension in the muscles at the back of the neck. Dizziness on looking up may be caused by pressure on some of the blood vessels that supply the brain.

## Diagnosis

Usually, your GP will be able to tell whether you have osteoarthritis after taking your history and examining you, as described on pages 9–10. Sometimes an X-ray will be needed. Osteoarthritis does not show up as abnormalities in blood tests (see pages 10–12).

## Treatment

The mainstays of treatment for osteoarthritis are:

- exercise

- reducing the strain on the affected joints and

- pain-killers when necessary.

The right kind of exercise will maintain movement and strengthen the muscles around a joint. This will stabilise the joint and protect it from strain.

If you are overweight, then losing some weight will help to take the strain off your lower back, knees, ankles and feet.

Pain-killers and sometimes anti-inflammatory drugs can relieve the pain and stiffness and allow you to benefit fully from an exercise programme.

For more detailed information on exercise, see pages 94–103 and for more information on treatment, turn to page 71.

## The outlook

The idea that disability caused by osteoarthritis is inevitable as we get older is old-fashioned. Although getting older is, of course, inevitable, disability is most definitely not inevitable. Modern medicine has a lot to offer and there is also a great deal that you can do to help yourself. If you learn to use your joints appropriately, you can remain healthy and active into old age. The way to do this is to avoid straining the joints but take plenty of the right sort of exercise, do not put on too much weight and use pain-killers when necessary.

Sometimes, joints become so damaged, painful and stiff that they can no longer work properly, in spite of regular exercise and pain-killers. The cartilage becomes thin and disappears completely and bone is moving on bone, instead of on cartilage. The joint may be painful all the time, even when it is held still and rested. Surgery to remove the worn-out joint and replace it with an artificial one may then be the answer.

Artificial hips and knees have been available for over 30 years and many thousands of these operations are performed every year, with a very high success rate. Indeed, joint replacement surgery is probably the greatest advance ever made in the treatment of arthritis! If you would like to know more, there is a separate book in the Family Doctor series, *Understanding Hip and Knee Arthritis Surgery,* which deals with these procedures.

## KEY POINTS

- Osteoarthritis affects most of us as we get older

- You will keep more active by avoiding strain to the joints, taking exercise, keeping your weight down and using pain-killers when the need arises

# Rheumatoid arthritis

## What is rheumatoid arthritis?

Rheumatoid arthritis is quite different from osteoarthritis. It is caused by an intense inflammation in the synovial joints and it can arise at any time from the teenage years onwards. It is more common in women and the peak age of onset is between 30 and 50.

Rheumatoid arthritis is the most common form of inflammatory arthritis and it affects one to two per cent of the population. Even so, it is much less common than osteoarthritis which affects almost all of us to some degree as we get older.

Rheumatoid arthritis should really be called 'rheumatoid disease' because not only the joints but other parts of the body may be affected – for example, the skin, lungs and eyes. As it is such a complex, widespread disease with many effects, rheumatoid arthritis is usually treated by hospital specialists – rheumatologists – and most sufferers attend hospital clinics.

## What's going on?

Rheumatoid arthritis is one of a group of conditions called 'autoimmune connective tissue diseases'. The other conditions in this group are much rarer. In all of these conditions, the body's immune system is overactive and appears to attack the body's own tissues. Something must trigger this process – for example, a virus or a toxin – but at the moment we do not know what.

A great deal of research is directed at finding the trigger with the hope of then developing a cure. But, although we do not have a cure at the present time, we do have drug treatments that are very effective at suppressing the over-activity of the immune system and keeping the process under control.

## A joint in rheumatoid arthritis

In rheumatoid arthritis the synovium, which lines the joint capsule, becomes swollen and inflamed. The inflammation can damage the cartilage and bone.

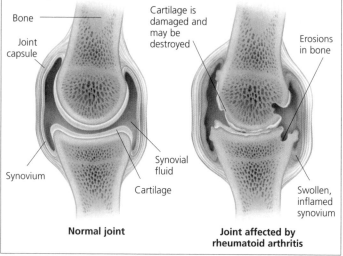

Bone

Joint capsule

Cartilage is damaged and may be destroyed

Erosions in bone

Synovium

Synovial fluid

Cartilage

Swollen, inflamed synovium

**Normal joint**

**Joint affected by rheumatoid arthritis**

We may not know the cause of rheumatoid arthritis but we do understand many of the changes that take place in the body tissues during the disease process. We know that the seat of the inflammation is the synovium, the slippery lining of joints, tendon sheaths and bursas. The synovium becomes swollen and thickened and may produce large amounts of synovial fluid. Cartilage and ligaments may be damaged and eventually the bone also may be damaged, forming cavities called 'erosions'.

In rare cases, the joint may eventually be destroyed. In severe cases, the inflammation may affect other tissues outside the joints, such as the eyes, skin and lungs.

## Symptoms

The symptoms of rheumatoid arthritis are varied and they may begin quite suddenly (see box).

### Symptoms in rheumatoid arthritis

- Many joints are affected at the same time with swelling, warmth and tenderness.
- The hands and feet are the most common joints involved, followed by the wrists, ankles, knees and shoulders, and neck.
- When the inflammation is active, fever, loss of appetite and weight loss are common.
- Many people feel tired and lacking in energy because they are anaemic.
- Severe stiffness first thing in the morning which tends to ease as the day progresses but may last for many hours.

In severe cases, morning stiffness seems to affect every joint in the body. Many people say that this stiffness and difficulty in getting going is more disabling than the pain. The inflammation may affect parts of the body outside the joints. Your eye may become red and sore and if this happens you will need to see an ophthalmologist. Your lungs may be affected and you should always report any increase in breathlessness to your doctor. Small blood vessels can become inflamed (a condition known as 'vasculitis'), causing rashes and sometimes ulcers.

## Rheumatoid nodules

Some people develop nodules under the skin at sites of friction, such as the feet, the backs of the heels, the backs of the hands and the elbows. The nodules are painless and, apart from being unsightly, do not usually cause trouble. Occasionally, they grow to a large size and interfere with the wearing of shoes. The nodules are easily removed by minor surgery but we try not to do this without good reason as they tend to recur.

## Later symptoms

Very occasionally, the symptoms of rheumatoid arthritis improve on their own after the first few weeks or months, but most people need treatment. Rheumatoid arthritis usually follows a pattern of 'remissions', followed by 'relapses' or 'flares'. Remissions are good periods when the symptoms are less troublesome and relapses are when the inflammation is more active.

The aim of treatment is to control the relapses and maintain, or prolong, the remissions. Often, remissions can last for many years.

## Who's who at the hospital clinic

- The consultant rheumatologist, who is in overall charge, selects and monitors the appropriate drugs, and coordinates the input of the other specialists. You may also sometimes see other members of the consultant's team, such as a specialist registrar or a senior house officer.
- The rheumatology nurse specialist will see you while your condition is in a stable phase to monitor your drug therapy. He or she is also a valuable contact for extra advice and information.
- The physiotherapist plays a vital role in relieving symptoms and preserving muscle strength and movement of affected joints. He or she may recommend splints for affected joints from time to time to protect them and maintain their correct position, and will also advise on the right sort of exercises for you to do at home.
- The occupational therapist is concerned with keeping you functioning as normally as possible and can advise on how to perform everyday activities most efficiently without straining the joints. He or she can also advise on aids and appliances.
- A podiatrist (as chiropodists are now known) may be needed if you develop foot problems, such as toe deformities, calluses and ulcers.
- The consultant orthopaedic surgeon will become involved if surgery, such as joint replacement, is being considered.
- Social workers can advise on the wide range of help and allowances that are available through the social services department of your local authority.

## Diagnosis

A detailed history, with a careful examination and some simple blood tests are usually all that are needed for an experienced doctor to make a diagnosis of rheumatoid arthritis. A full blood count will show whether you are anaemic (a reduced number of red blood cells, common in rheumatoid arthritis) and an erythrocyte sedimentation rate (ESR) will show whether inflammation is present.

A test for rheumatoid factor (see page 12) may help in the diagnosis. X-rays often appear normal in the early stages of the disease but they should be taken so that they can be used as a baseline against which to compare later X-rays. A chest X-ray and X-rays of the hands and feet are the most useful.

## Treatment

The aims underlying treatment for rheumatoid arthritis are to:

● relieve symptoms

● preserve muscle strength and joint movement

● protect the joints from further damage

● help the individual to lead as normal a life as possible.

At the hospital clinic, you will meet a number of specialists, each of whom can help in a different way (see page 25).

## Drug treatments

There are several different types of drug used to treat rheumatoid arthritis. First and very important are non-steroidal anti-inflammatory drugs (NSAIDs) and analgesics (simple pain-killers). They are dealt with in the section on drugs on page 71 but, briefly, anti-inflammatory drugs reduce pain, stiffness and swelling, whereas analgesics provide added pain relief if this is necessary. Although these drugs can help the symptoms of rheumatoid arthritis, they do not have any effect on the long-term progression of the disease.

This is the role of the second and equally important group of drugs that help to prevent joint damage. The drugs in this group are methotrexate, sulfasalazine, azathioprine, leflunomide (Arava), gold salts, penicillamine and hydroxychloroquine. Methotrexate and sulfasalazine appear to be the most effective and so these are the DMARDs that are most often used.

Each has been shown to improve the long-term outcome in people with rheumatoid arthritis and they are known collectively as 'disease-modifying anti-rheumatoid drugs' or 'DMARDs' (pronounced 'deemards') (see box on page 28). These drugs are chemically very different from each other – we do not yet know in detail how they work but they have some common features.

Several new DMARDs work directly on the immune system. Examples are etanercept (Enbrel), infliximab (Remicade), adalimumab (Humira) and rituximab (MabThera). As a group, they are known as 'biologics' or 'biological agents'. They are powerful drugs that are given by injection and need to be closely monitored. Long-term effects are not yet clear so they are reserved for people with severe arthritis who have not been helped by other DMARDs. But these drugs can have a dramatic effect in some people and they are being much more widely used. Two of the drugs, etanercept

## About DMARDs

- All DMARDs take a long time to take effect – eight to twelve weeks – and they need to be taken long term for the effect to be maintained. In other words, you do not stop taking them as soon as you feel better!

- Not all DMARDs are effective in all individuals, so if the first one that you try does not help then your rheumatologist may suggest that you try a different one, or perhaps a combination of drugs.

- All DMARDs have side effects but, in general, these can be picked up very early by blood tests and urine tests, before any harm is done. So anyone taking these drugs will need to have regular tests to monitor for problems. You should be given a booklet by your rheumatologist or hospital pharmacist to record the results of these tests.

and adalimumab, can be given by injections under the skin. People taking these drugs (or their relative or carer) can be taught to give the injections at home, making the treatment much more convenient.

Steroids can be useful in treating rheumatoid arthritis because they have a powerful anti-inflammatory action. They may be given as a course of tablets or by injection into particularly troublesome joints from time to time.

There is more about this and other types of treatment in the chapter starting on page 71.

## The outlook

If it is not treated, rheumatoid arthritis goes through

relapses (flares) and remissions. Flares may be triggered by illness, such as influenza, or even by stress, such as bereavement. If the flares are frequent and severe, then damage to joints accumulates and they may be destroyed.

Severe disease affecting the joints and other body tissues is fortunately rare. When first told the diagnosis, many people are shocked and upset and a common question is 'Will I be in a wheelchair, doctor?'. They fear that rheumatoid arthritis automatically means immobility, disability and dependency. This is no longer true.

Many sufferers have only mild arthritis and symptoms of pain and stiffness are kept at bay with tablets and exercise. Even those with more extensive problems can, with the right help, lead almost normal lives with jobs and families.

## KEY POINTS

- Rheumatoid arthritis causes joints to become inflamed – it is very different to osteoarthritis

- A lot of help is available for people with rheumatoid arthritis, mostly from specialists at the hospital clinic

# Gout

## Who gets gout?

There is a popular belief that only middle-aged, overweight men who eat and drink too much suffer from gout. This is a myth – gout can attack young men in their twenties and also women, although it is very unusual in women and occurs mainly after the menopause. One survey of general practice patients found that gout affects 6 in every 1,000 men and 1 in every 1,000 women in the UK.

## What's going on?

An attack of gout is caused by uric acid suddenly forming crystals inside a joint, causing intense inflammation with pain, redness and swelling. Uric acid is produced when purines, which are chemicals present within all living cells, are broken down. Purines are produced by the body itself and are also found in many foods. People prone to gout have an inherited tendency to produce a lot of uric acid. High levels accumulate in the bloodstream and are deposited in the body's tissues.

Common sites are the joints, the kidneys and the skin over the tops of the ears, hands and elbows. If the kidneys are affected, then they do not work as well as they should at excreting the uric acid in the urine and the levels become even higher. Uric acid deposits under the skin appear as whitish lumps, called 'tophi'. They may ulcerate and discharge material that looks like toothpaste. It is not always clear what causes the uric acid suddenly to form crystals in the joints and set off inflammation, but a common trigger is minor injury to the joint.

## Symptoms

A typical attack of gout is easily recognisable (see below).

### What happens during an attack of gout

- At first, there is only minor discomfort but, within a matter of hours, the joint is swollen, hot, red and extremely painful.
- The pain is so severe that wearing shoes is out of the question, and you may not even be able to bear the touch of a bedsheet.
- Even with no treatment, the attack subsides completely within a few days, and always within a week.
- Attacks may recur, although sometimes not until months or years later.
- In 70 per cent of people, the knuckle joint of the big toe is the first joint, and often the only joint, to be affected, although symptoms can develop in any joint.

## Diagnosis

Often your doctor will be able to recognise that you have gout from your symptoms and the appearance of the affected joint. You will need to have blood tests to measure the amount of uric acid in your bloodstream and to check whether your kidneys have been affected. A sample of fluid may sometimes be taken from an acutely inflamed joint with a fine needle and syringe.

Examination of the fluid under a special polarising microscope will show crystals of uric acid. This test will distinguish between gout and a condition called 'pseudogout'. In pseudogout, the symptoms of an acute attack may mimic gout but the crystals responsible are calcium pyrophosphate. Pseudogout occurs in elderly people with osteoarthritis and is not usually inherited.

## Treatment

Non-steroidal anti-inflammatory drugs are very effective and can shorten an attack if they are taken right at the beginning. Before these drugs became available, the traditional treatment for an attack of gout was a drug called colchicine, derived from the autumn crocus.

Colchicine is still used and it is also very effective, although it can cause troublesome diarrhoea in some people. In fact, both anti-inflammatory drugs and colchicine are so effective if taken early that people who have frequent attacks of gout are well advised to keep a supply in the medicine cabinet, so that they can take it at the first sign of trouble.

# Diagnosing gout as a cause of joint pain

An attack of gout is caused by uric acid suddenly forming crystals within a joint, causing intense inflammation with pain, redness and swelling.

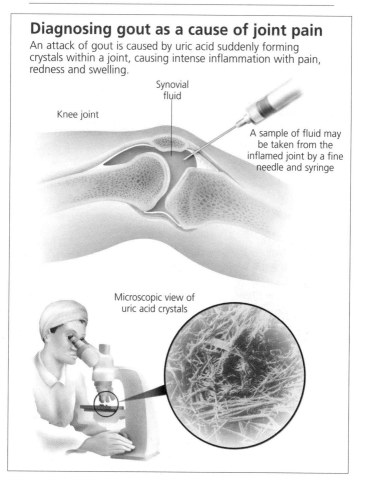

Synovial fluid

Knee joint

A sample of fluid may be taken from the inflamed joint by a fine needle and syringe

Microscopic view of uric acid crystals

## Looking ahead

If you still get frequent attacks, say more than three times a year, despite these measures, your doctor may suggest that you take drugs to lower the level of uric acid in your body. The main one is allopurinol which, taken daily as tablets, blocks the chemical pathway leading to uric acid production.

## Help yourself to avoid gout

- Drink plenty of clear dilute fluids (water or cordial), at least three litres a day, especially in hot weather and when you're on holiday, because an attack is more likely if you become dehydrated.

- Reduce your weight so that it is within the normal range for your height (see page 108).

- Keep your alcohol consumption within recommended levels – 21 units a week for a man and 14 for a woman. A unit is half a pint of beer, a small glass of wine or a single measure of spirits.

- Cut down on food and drink containing high levels of purines; these include high-protein foods such as red meat and pulses, offal (liver and kidneys), sardines and anchovies. It is better to eat meals based around complex carbohydrates, such as pasta. If you are concerned about what you should be eating, ask to see a dietitian.

- Avoid taking aspirin, which stops the kidneys from excreting uric acid; take paracetamol instead for minor aches and pains.

The uric acid deposits in the body tissues are then slowly removed into the urine and so leave the body. This effect takes place slowly, and you will still be prone to attacks of gout while the level of uric acid in your body remains high. Other drugs, less commonly used, work by making the kidneys more effective at excreting uric acid.

When you first start taking any of these long-term treatments, there is a temporarily increased risk of having an attack of gout, so you will usually be advised to take an anti-inflammatory drug at the same time for the first three months. Once you are on the long-term preventive treatment, you will probably have to continue with it indefinitely.

**KEY POINTS**

■ Gout attacks are very painful but they get better within a few days, even without treatment

■ If attacks are frequent, then you may need to take tablets every day to reduce the level of uric acid in your body

# Other forms of inflammatory arthritis

Osteoarthritis, rheumatoid arthritis and gout are the most common forms of arthritis but there are several other types that are also important, although they are much rarer. Some of these forms of arthritis develop in people with other conditions – the arthritis may form a major part of the disease or be a relatively minor problem. In these forms of arthritis, the joints are inflamed, that is, like rheumatoid arthritis, they are forms of inflammatory arthritis.

## Ankylosing spondylitis

This condition causes inflammation of the joints in the spine, including the sacroiliac joints which link the spine to the pelvis, and the hips are also sometimes affected. It is three times more common in men than in women and it usually develops between the ages of 20 and 40. The risk is 10 to 20 times higher for those who have a parent, brother or sister with the condition.

Ankylosing spondylitis is closely linked with an inherited factor known as tissue type HLA-B27. Only about 8 per cent of the population have HLA-B27, but 95 per cent of ankylosing spondylitis sufferers carry this tissue type.

## Symptoms of ankylosing spondylitis

The main symptom is pain and stiffness in the lower back and hips, which is much worse in the mornings when it often lasts for several hours. The spine loosens up with activity and exercise but the stiffness recurs the following morning. Without treatment, the stiffness may spread to involve the whole spine, including the neck.

A programme of daily exercises and regular review by a physiotherapist are vital to maintain the flexibility of the spine. Without regular exercise, the spine, over time, becomes curved and fixed. Drugs can ease the pain and the subjective feeling of stiffness, but they cannot take the place of exercise in maintaining movement.

Occasionally, other joints may be affected, and pain under the heel (plantar fasciitis, see page 67) can be troublesome. Sufferers may occasionally develop inflammation of the eye with red, painful watering and blurred vision. This requires urgent treatment from an ophthalmologist.

There are a number of other conditions that are similar to ankylosing spondylitis. The whole group is known medically as 'spondyloarthritis'. These other conditions are described below.

## Reactive arthritis (sometimes called Reiter's syndrome)

This develops in some people after an infection of the bowel or urogenital system. A small number of joints, usually a knee or an ankle or both, become very swollen and painful. The joints are not infected but the inflammation develops as a result of the body's reaction to the infection – hence the term 'reactive arthritis'. Back pain, eye inflammation and a rash on the soles of the feet can also occur.

## Inflammatory bowel disease, particularly ulcerative colitis

This can occasionally cause joint inflammation, in a pattern similar to ankylosing spondylitis but also affecting large joints such as hips, knees or ankles.

## Psoriatic arthritis

Psoriasis is a very common skin condition which affects about two per cent of the population. A small proportion of these – less than 10 per cent – develop inflammatory arthritis. The joint problems may develop even though the psoriasis is mild and, occasionally, they may appear before any skin changes.

On the other hand, psoriasis sufferers with severe skin disease may never have joint problems. Psoriatic arthritis is a form of spondyloarthritis but in severe cases it can be difficult to distinguish it from rheumatoid arthritis as it often affects the small joints of the hands and feet, as well as the large joints.

## Symptoms of psoriatic arthritis

Unlike rheumatoid arthritis, psoriatic arthritis may occur unevenly. In other words, one hand may be affected but not the other. Eight of ten people with psoriatic arthritis will notice that psoriasis affects their nails, so that they become pitted and chalky.

Around a third of people experience lower back pain as a result of inflammation in their sacroiliac joints, something that rarely happens in rheumatoid arthritis. Mild cases are treated with exercise and anti-inflammatory drugs. For severe cases, the drug treatment is similar to that for rheumatoid arthritis (see page 71).

## Arthritis in children

Children may develop painful and swollen joints, usually after a viral infection or an injury, and the condition usually settles quickly. Arthritis that lasts for more than 12 weeks is unusual and may be caused by chronic inflammation. This condition is called 'juvenile idiopathic arthritis' (idiopathic means that we do not know the cause of the arthritis). In the UK it affects around 12,000 children of all ages. The number of joints affected varies from one individual to another. Some children develop eye inflammation and some children may be ill with a fever and a rash.

All children with arthritis need specialist care by a hospital team, working together with their parents and teachers to ensure that the child can live as normal a life as possible.

Many children grow out of the condition in a few years, but a few have persistent problems as they grow up and a small number develop an adult form of the condition.

## KEY POINTS

- There are several types of inflammatory arthritis – rheumatoid arthritis is the most common

- Children and young people can develop inflammatory arthritis and they need specialist care from a hospital clinic

# Other inflammatory conditions

Some other conditions, unrelated to spondyloarthritis, can cause inflammation associated with mild arthritis. The inflammation is more widespread and, as well as the joints, it affects tissues elsewhere in the body. The Arthritis Research Campaign (see Useful addresses on page 113) publishes free information leaflets on all these conditions.

## Systemic lupus erythematosus

Systemic lupus erythematosus (SLE or lupus) is a member of a group of conditions called 'connective tissue diseases' (connective tissue supports and connects other body parts). SLE is similar to rheumatoid arthritis in that it is an autoimmune disease (see page 22) but it is much rarer and the arthritis is usually much less severe. Around 90 per cent of those affected are young women between the ages of 20 and 40, and women of African–Caribbean origin are particularly susceptible.

## Symptoms of SLE

- Painful, swollen joints, particularly in the hands

- Feeling generally unwell and feverish

- Rash on the face, particularly in response to sunlight

- Thinning of the hair.

Most people with SLE have mild disease which comes and goes, affecting only their joints and skin and causing mild anaemia. A few develop severe inflammation of the internal organs, such as the kidneys, lungs and nervous system, and some women suffer repeated miscarriages of pregnancy. SLE responds very well to steroids but, in cases of severe disease, other drugs that suppress the immune system may also be needed.

## Polymyositis

Polymyositis is also a connective tissue disorder, rarer than SLE. It mainly affects the muscles which become inflamed and very weak. In the related condition of dermatomyositis, the skin is also affected. Both conditions respond to steroids which may need to be used in large doses for a time.

## Polymyalgia rheumatica

Polymyalgia rheumatica (PMR) is quite a common condition. It affects older people and is very rare in anyone younger than 50. It is not related to the connective tissue diseases.

'Polymyalgia' literally means 'pain in many muscles' but the condition appears to result from inflammation in the joints of the shoulder girdle and pelvic girdle, rather than in the muscles.

## Symptoms of PMR

- Severe pain and stiffness around the shoulders and hips, which is noticeably much worse in the mornings

- Difficulty turning over in bed at night without help

- Feeling generally unwell and tired, sometimes feverish

- Loss of weight

- Depression.

## Diagnosis of PMR

Your doctor will often be able to diagnose the condition from the symptoms that you describe and the results of a blood test to measure the erythrocyte sedimentation rate (ESR). The ESR is usually very high in polymyalgia (see page 11), indicating the presence of inflammation.

## Treatment of PMR

Steroids taken by mouth or by injection have a dramatic effect and within 24 hours you should feel almost back to normal. The steroids should not be stopped too quickly as you may need to stay on treatment for many months (occasionally, for several years) to allow the polymyalgia to settle down.

For more about treatments see 'Treating arthritis and rheumatism' on page 71.

## KEY POINTS

- Some rare conditions cause inflammation in many areas of the body, including the joints; these are best treated with steroids, which are powerful anti-inflammatory drugs

# Non-inflammatory conditions

**Fibromyalgia**

Fibromyalgia is often confused with polymyalgia (see page 42) but in fibromyalgia there is no sign of inflammation. People with fibromyalgia are often worried that they have arthritis or some other serious disease but this is almost never the case. Blood tests and X-rays are normal.

Most people with fibromyalgia are women in their middle years – and in some cases the symptoms seem to be triggered by bereavement or stress and they are often associated with poor sleep (see below). It can be difficult to decide whether the chronic pain of the condition led to the symptoms of tiredness, fatigue and poor sleep, or whether insufficient sleep or poor quality sleep is actually the root cause of the problem.

## Symptoms of fibromyalgia

- Widespread pain and tenderness, particularly across the shoulders, back, elbows and knees

- Although the joints and soft tissues are tender, they are not swollen

- The muscles and joints may feel stiff in the mornings but this disappears quickly once you get up

- Low spirits or depression

- Poor sleep

- Lack of energy.

**Treatment**

Your doctor may prescribe medication to lift depression and help you to sleep more soundly if necessary. Remaining as active and mobile as possible will help. If you rest a lot, you may feel worse as you will become unfit and more tired and your muscles will become weaker and more susceptible to injury. Regular exercise can also help to clear your mind and improve the quality of your sleep. You can help yourself with some other simple lifestyle changes (see box below) in addition to any treatment provided by your GP.

### Self-help tips for fibromyalgia

- Don't drink coffee or other caffeine-containing drinks in the evening because they may disturb your sleep
- Consider relaxation classes
- Try to deal with any major sources of stress in your daily life
- Keep as active as possible, and consider taking up some gentle, regular exercise such as swimming or brisk walking

## Hypermobility

This is not actually a disease but it may be a cause of very painful joints in young people. People come in all shapes and sizes and there is a similar variation in joint flexibility. Some people normally have rather stiff joints whereas, at the other extreme, some have very supple, mobile joints and are often called 'double-jointed'. If you are one of these people, you may be able to bend over with your knees straight and put your hands flat on the floor in front of you when most of us struggle just to touch our toes. Your elbows and knees may bend backwards and your fingers may turn up when you hold them outstretched. If you can do this, you may have 'hypermobility syndrome'.

Hypermobility represents the supple end of the normal spectrum of joint mobility. A small number of people with extremely mobile joints suffer recurrent dislocations and their joints are easily damaged but most people with hypermobility have it in a mild form. Very supple joints are easily strained by everyday activities and people with painful, hypermobile joints

### Self-help tips for hypermobile joints

- Take care not to strain your joints
- Take regular exercise to build up your muscles – well-toned muscles will help to support your joints and protect them from strain
- Avoid exercises or activities that overstretch the joints, such as ballet and gymnastics
- Most important of all, resist the temptation to perform 'party tricks' to show off your mobile joints

## Hypermobility

Hypermobility represents the supple end of the normal spectrum of joint mobility.

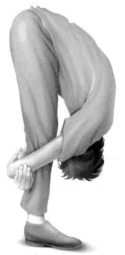

may worry that they have arthritis although this is unlikely to be the case. A few simple measures will help to keep the pain under control (see page 47).

## Neck and back problems
### Back pain

Low back pain, or lumbago, is very common: 80 per cent of the population experience it at some time in their lives. Most back pain is 'non-specific' or 'mechanical' – in other words, it results from some minor physical problem in the complex structure of the back, such as a strained muscle, ligament or tendon, which will heal on its own in time. Serious causes of back pain are very rare indeed. Surprisingly, the severity of the pain is not a good guide to the seriousness of the cause and in fact the most severe pains are usually non-specific and should heal in their own time.

Correcting poor posture, taking care with lifting and carrying, and performing regular exercise can all help. Much useful information about the spine can be found in the book *Understanding Back Pain* in the Family Doctor series.

## Sciatica

Sometimes pain is felt in one of the legs as well as in the back. Sciatica, which is caused by pressure on a nerve by a disc in the spine, is one cause and the leg pain may be accompanied by tingling, pins and needles or numbness. Although this is often referred to as a 'slipped disc', discs do not actually slip in and out. A more correct name is 'prolapsed disc' or 'ruptured disc'. Discs are filled with a jelly which acts as a cushion between the bones of the spinal column. When a disc ruptures, or tears, some of this jelly squirts out and can irritate a nearby nerve, causing severe pain down the leg (see diagram on page 50).

### Treatment

With pain-killers, a few days' rest, and then gentle exercise and physiotherapy, the tear heals, the disc material is absorbed and the pressure on the nerve is relieved. It is important to keep as mobile as the pain permits, although initially a day or two of bed rest may be necessary if the pain is severe. Most people get completely better in a few weeks, but in a small number of people, symptoms do not get better with pain-killers and physiotherapy and they may need surgery to remove the disc material.

# Back pain caused by prolapsed disc

Sometimes pain is felt in one of the legs as well as in the back. This may be caused by a prolapsed disc in the spine.

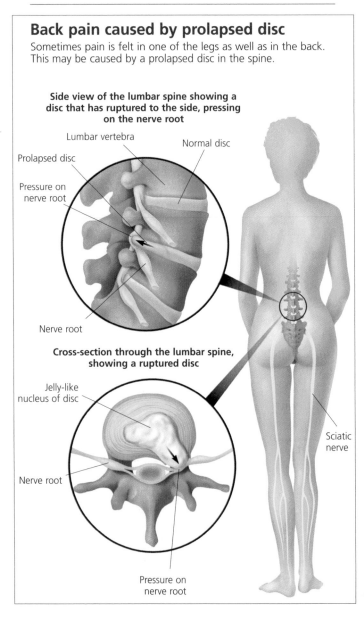

**Side view of the lumbar spine showing a disc that has ruptured to the side, pressing on the nerve root**

Lumbar vertebra

Normal disc

Prolapsed disc

Pressure on nerve root

Nerve root

**Cross-section through the lumbar spine, showing a ruptured disc**

Jelly-like nucleus of disc

Nerve root

Pressure on nerve root

Sciatic nerve

## Neck pain

Pain in the neck is probably as common as pain in the back and often has similar causes, although a ruptured disc is much less common in the neck than in the lower back. Poor posture is a common culprit. Many people hunch their shoulders and allow their head to poke forwards. The head is very heavy (as heavy as a bucket of water) and, to stop the head from flopping onto the chest, the muscles at the back of the neck have to work hard to hold the head up.

Eventually, this chronic contraction, or tension, causes aching pain and stiffness in the trapezius muscles across the shoulders, and up the neck to the back of the head. It can even cause severe headaches (tension headaches) felt across the forehead and behind the eyes.

### Treatment

Treatment involves understanding the problem, correcting the posture and performing regular simple exercises to loosen the muscles and keep the neck supple.

## Arthritis of the spine

Degenerative arthritis, or spondylosis, of the spine is extremely common. If an X-ray was taken of the spine of everyone over the age of 50, almost all of them would show degenerative changes. But not all of these people have back pain and, of those who do, the pain often comes and goes. So there is no clear relationship between X-ray changes and symptoms. Regardless of whether there are degenerative changes on the X-ray, most episodes of back pain will get better with pain-killers and a few days' rest, followed by gentle exercise and then getting back to normal activities. It is important to keep as mobile as the pain permits, although initially a day or two of bed rest may be necessary if the pain is severe. But if the back pain lasts longer than a week and you find it difficult to get back to work, then you should consult your doctor.

Another form of arthritis that affects the spine is ankylosing spondylitis. This is a rare form of inflammatory arthritis and it has been described earlier (see page 36).

## Osteoporosis

In older people, especially women, pain in the upper back may be the result of osteoporosis ('thinning of

## Osteoporosis

In osteoporosis, the bones become thinner and weaker. Vertebrae may collapse, causing the back to become rounded.

Fracture of osteoporotic vertebra, causing wedging with loss of anterior height the bones'). Everyone loses calcium from their bones as they get older, especially women after the menopause. The process is usually very slow, but there may come a point when the bones have lost so much calcium that they are thin and prone to fracture. The vertebrae in the upper back may become distorted so that the back becomes very rounded ('dowager's hump'). There may be chronic pain, or episodes of acute pain, when a single bone collapses slightly. If you think that you may have osteoporosis, consult your doctor.

There are now treatments available that can slow down the loss of calcium from the bones and even make them a little stronger. You can help by giving up smoking, making sure that your diet has plenty of calcium and taking regular exercise – even a brisk walk for half an hour three times a week can make a difference.

Much more detailed information about osteoporosis is contained in the book *Understanding Osteoporosis* in the Family Doctor series, or can be obtained from the National Osteoporosis Society (see Useful addresses, page 119).

## Problems in and around individual joints

'Soft-tissue rheumatism' is the term used to describe a group of painful conditions that are caused by problems with the soft tissues around joints, rather than problems with the joints themselves. Tendons, which join muscles to bone, ligaments, which join bones together, and bursas can all be responsible.

The general principles of treatment of these conditions involve steroid injections to settle the pain and inflammation in the acute phase, a splint to rest the painful area and, most important of all, recognising what activity caused the problem and either avoiding the activity altogether or changing the way that it is done. If this aspect of the treatment is neglected, then there is a risk that the problem will recur. Many sports injuries fall into this category.

## Shoulder pain

Pain felt around the shoulder can sometimes be caused by neck problems. This is particularly true if the pain is felt on top of the shoulder in the large trapezius muscle that runs between the shoulder joint proper and the neck.

Pain arising from the shoulder joint itself is often felt in the upper arm rather than over the point of the shoulder. Common causes are frozen shoulder (also known as 'adhesive capsulitis') and tendinitis.

### Frozen shoulder

This mainly affects older people and is rare under the age of 50. The symptoms usually begin suddenly and may follow a minor injury, such as a knock or a fall, although the injury may be so minor as to be forgotten. Occasionally, frozen shoulder can follow an attack of shingles or even a heart attack.

We do not know what causes frozen shoulder but we do know that the capsule surrounding the joint becomes thickened and inflamed, causing pain. The inflamed capsule is 'sticky' and adhesions form between the capsule and the bones, restricting the movement of the joint.

### Symptoms of frozen shoulder

- Constant pain which can be very severe, even when the shoulder is held still.

- Difficulty sleeping because of the pain – it may also be impossible to lie on the affected side.

- Severe stiffness, which may make it very difficult to reach up to a shelf or into a back pocket or, in some cases, to move the joint at all.

**Treatment**

Even without treatment, the pain of a frozen shoulder will usually settle within 18 months, but most people don't want to wait that long! When the shoulder is intensely painful, the most effective treatment is steroid injection into the joint. This relieves the pain, although sometimes more than one injection is needed.

The other, equally important, aspect of treatment is regular exercise to bring back the range of movement

## Exercises for frozen shoulder

- Stand up and lean your trunk slightly over towards the side of the affected shoulder, so that your arm hangs away from your body. Swing the arm gently backwards and forwards, keeping your elbow straight and avoid shrugging your shoulder as you swing. Swing backwards and forwards 10 times and repeat the whole exercise several times a day.

- Lean forwards and gently swing your arm from side to side across your body, moving the shoulder joint in a different direction, then swing the arm in a circular movement. As the shoulder becomes freer, you will find that you can swing further and further and in ever larger circles.

- Reach behind your waist with your good arm and grasp the wrist of the arm with the frozen shoulder. Gently pull the arm behind your back, being careful not to force the movement.

and prevent the shoulder becoming stiff and stuck once the pain has gone.

When doing the exercises described in the box on page 55, don't stretch or move beyond the point where you feel slight pain. Forcing your shoulder through a wider range of movement will just make the problem worse. But with careful attention to regular exercise, you should regain useful movement in your shoulder, although it may always remain slightly restricted compared with your normal side.

## Shoulder tendinitis

Inflammation of the tendons or the sheaths containing them is a common cause of shoulder pain. A normal shoulder has an enormous range of movement – you can put your arms up above your head, bring them out to the sides and swing them up behind your back.

This is a legacy from our evolutionary ancestors who needed this range of movement to swing through trees. Unfortunately, it means that the tendons of the shoulder are easily damaged and subject to wear. They can fray and bleed a little, leading to inflammation. This causes pain which is always worse when the shoulder is moved and less severe at rest.

### Treatment

Injection of steroid into the area around the inflamed tendon can be very effective. After a couple of days, you can start on a gentle programme of exercise to restore normal movement to your shoulder. The exercises are likely to be similar to those for frozen shoulder (see page 55), but your doctor or physiotherapist will explain precisely what you need to do.

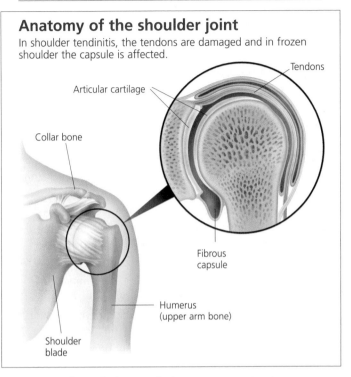

## Anatomy of the shoulder joint

In shoulder tendinitis, the tendons are damaged and in frozen shoulder the capsule is affected.

Tendons

Articular cartilage

Collar bone

Fibrous capsule

Humerus
(upper arm bone)

Shoulder blade

Once the pain has settled, you must resist the temptation to perform heavy lifting and you should pace any work that is heavy on the shoulders, such as cleaning windows, digging in the garden and using a vacuum cleaner.

You should also beware the 'perils of the plastic carrier bag'! Plastic shopping bags are very strong and have small handles. They can be loaded up with heavy shopping and the small handles mean that the bags have to be carried with the arms held vertically downwards. The weight drags on the elbows and shoulders and also the neck, straining the tissues and causing pain.

Heavy shopping should ideally be carried in a trolley on wheels. If this is not possible (trolleys can be difficult to take on and off the bus), then small amounts of shopping can be carried in a stiff basket with a wide handle, carried over the forearm. Most of the weight of the basket can then be carried on the hip avoiding undue strain on the the arms.

## Tennis elbow and golfer's elbow

These conditions cause pain at the points at which the tendon attaches to the bone around the elbow. Tennis elbow causes pain on the outer side of the elbow, where the extensor muscles on the outer side of the forearm are attached (see diagram opposite). These muscles bend the wrist back and straighten the fingers. Golfer's elbow is much less common and causes pain on the inner side of the elbow, at the attachment of the flexor muscles which bend the wrist forwards and flex the fingers.

Both conditions were first described in sportsmen but most sufferers develop them as a result of everyday activities, such as repeated heavy lifting, pushing and pulling. Sometimes a single episode of awkward lifting, such as lifting a heavy case down from an overhead locker, may be the trigger. The lifting need not be heavy: office workers who repeatedly pull files out of tight, over-stuffed cabinets are also at risk.

### Treatment

A steroid injection into the painful area is usually helpful. Physiotherapy may also be beneficial. But most important is to work out what caused the problem in the first place and avoid the activity in future, otherwise the symptoms may recur and can become chronic.

## Tennis elbow

Right arm seen from the right side. When the extensor muscle contracts, to bend the wrist back, the muscle pulls on the bone. This causes pain if the area is inflamed, as in 'tennis elbow'.

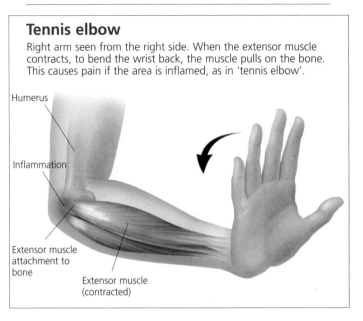

Humerus

Inflammation

Extensor muscle attachment to bone

Extensor muscle (contracted)

## Overuse syndrome (repetitive strain injury, RSI)

There has been much discussion in the courts (where sufferers have claimed compensation from their employers) as to whether this condition really exists, but most doctors agree that it does.

Like many other soft-tissue problems, this condition is triggered by misuse or overuse of the affected part of the body. It is also called 'upper limb syndrome' and affects the neck, shoulders, arms and hands of keyboard workers and other people who continually repeat the same tasks and movements in their work. In fact, people employed to pluck chickens were the first group in whom the condition was identified.

The pain is not confined to any one area but is most severe in the backs of the hands and forearms, and is

## Anatomy of the hand and wrist

The wrist and hand contain very many bones.

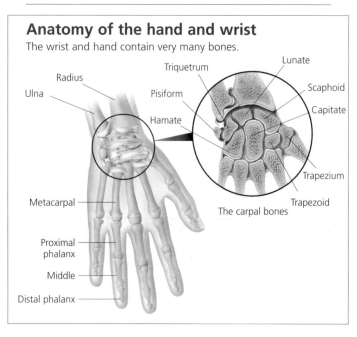

Radius

Ulna

Triquetrum

Pisiform

Hamate

Lunate

Scaphoid

Capitate

Trapezium

Trapezoid

The carpal bones

Metacarpal

Proximal phalanx

Middle

Distal phalanx

clearly related to work. At the beginning, it may come on only towards the end of a busy day. If left untreated, it can progress and then the time between starting work and developing the pain gets shorter.

In severe cases, there is some pain all the time, even when not at work, and normal daily activities outside work may also trigger pain.

### Treatment

If the symptoms have been neglected and the condition has been allowed to become severe and chronic, treatment is difficult and not always successful. It is vital to act promptly as soon as you suspect that you may be developing problems. Look very carefully at the nature of your work and your workstation. Physiotherapists and occupational therapists are experts in these assessments but there are a number of things that you can change yourself: see the self-help tips on pages 62–3. Discuss the situation with your employers and see your GP or the company's occupational health doctor, if there is one.

Although most cases of overuse syndrome occur as a result of practices at work, if you use a computer (or other equipment, such as a sewing machine or DIY tools) a lot at home, you can develop exactly the same problems. The principles of pacing, technique, proper positioning and posture still apply. With careful attention to these principles, most people are able to continue with their work.

## Carpal tunnel syndrome

In this very common condition, there is pressure on the median nerve as it passes through the wrist (see diagram on page 64). The bones of the wrist (the carpal bones) are arranged in a horseshoe shape. The free ends of the horseshoe are joined together by a tough piece of tissue, forming a narrow tunnel through which the median nerve passes.

Any swelling of the tissues in the area can cause pressure on the nerve and irritate it. Signals sent from the median nerve to the brain are interpreted as coming from the area supplied by this nerve – that is, from the hand (see below). Carpal tunnel syndrome can be caused by fluid retention, such as occurs in pregnancy or when the thyroid gland is underactive, or be a symptom of rheumatoid arthritis, but very often no underlying cause is identified.

## Self-help tips to avoid RSI

- **Alternate your work.** Split it up and mix different tasks – instead of spending two whole days typing and then two days filing, alternate every few hours.

- **Take regular breaks.** If your job involves mainly one activity such as using a computer, then it is vitally important that you take regular breaks. Every hour, stand up, stretch your legs, lift your arms above your head, and open and close your hands. Focus on distant objects through the window to rest your eyes. This takes only a couple of minutes but will make all the difference to how long you can work without discomfort.

- **Improve your technique.** If you're a keyboard worker and can't touch-type, it is worth learning to do so because this allows you to spread the work of typing over all your fingers and thumbs and means that you can hold your head up instead of looking down at the keyboard.

- **Make sure that your equipment and furniture are properly positioned.** You should have a height-adjustable chair on wheels, with a backrest and without arms so that you can sit close up to your desk. Your computer screen and keyboard should be placed directly in front of you – just a few inches to one side will place strain on your arms and neck. The screen should be slightly lower than your sight-line – any lower and you will hunch your shoulders and lean forward, any higher and you will crane your neck. All other equipment that you use regularly, such as the telephone, should be placed close to you so that you are not continually reaching across the desk.

## Self-help tips to avoid RSI (contd)

- **Pay attention to your posture.** The best-designed equipment will do nothing for you if it is not used properly. Adjust the height of your chair so that your feet are comfortably placed on the floor or on a foot-rest and your forearms rest comfortably on the desk. Don't slouch in the chair but sit up straight, preserving the curve in your lower back. Sit close to your desk so that your hands rest on the keyboard without stretching your arms forward. Your shoulders should be relaxed, your upper arms should hang vertically downwards and your forearms should be held at right angles when typing.

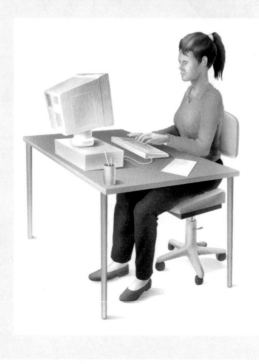

## Carpal tunnel syndrome

Carpal tunnel syndrome is caused by pressure on the median nerve as it passes through the carpal tunnel – which is formed by the bones of the wrist and the ligaments over them.

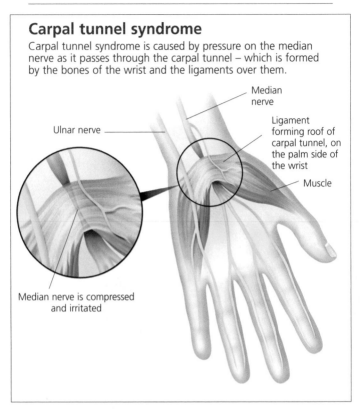

Median nerve

Ligament forming roof of carpal tunnel, on the palm side of the wrist

Muscle

Ulnar nerve

Median nerve is compressed and irritated

## Symptoms of carpal tunnel syndrome

- Numbness, tingling or pain in the hand, worse in the thumb, index and middle fingers.

- Symptoms are much worse during the night or first thing in the morning and may disappear completely during the day.

- Rubbing or shaking the hand eases the pain and tingling.

## Treatment

The priority is to relieve the pressure on the nerve, which increases when your wrist is bent forwards and reduces when it is bent back. A simple splint worn around your wrist at night to stop it bending forward may be enough to solve the problem; your GP or a physiotherapist can supply one for you. You can also help yourself by making sure that your wrists are not bent forwards when you are sitting with your hands in your lap or with your arms folded. If this does not work, then an injection of steroid into the carpal tunnel can shrink the tissues enough to relieve the pressure.

If this is not effective either, a simple operation under local anaesthetic will relieve the pressure on the nerve.

## Thumb tendinitis (de Quervain's tenosynovitis)

In this condition, the pain arises from the tendons that work the thumb. Tendons run inside a lubricated sheath but, when they become inflamed, movement causes the surfaces to grate against each other (see diagram on page 66). The base of the thumb and the lower end of the forearm become painful, and the area may be tender and even swollen. Parents who lift their young children by holding them under the armpits are particularly prone to this complaint; so are restaurant staff who carry heavy plates of food in each hand with the weight balanced by the thumb.

Osteoarthritis of the joint at the base of the thumb, where it is attached to the wrist, can cause similar symptoms.

## Treatment

Thumb tendinitis usually responds very well to a steroid

## Thumb tendinitis

Tendons run inside a lubricated sheath but, when they become inflamed, movement causes the surfaces to grate against each other resulting in pain.

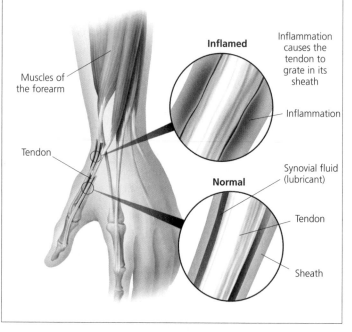

Muscles of the forearm

Tendon

**Inflamed**

Inflammation causes the tendon to grate in its sheath

Inflammation

Synovial fluid (lubricant)

**Normal**

Tendon

Sheath

injection into the sheath of the tendon together with a splint to rest the thumb. It is also very important to identify the activity that caused the problem and avoid it.

## Trigger finger

Make a fist and then straighten your fingers. If one finger lags behind the others, at first refusing to straighten and then suddenly straightening with a 'click', you have trigger finger. The condition is the result of a nodule that develops on the tendon as it runs through the palm of the hand. The nodule catches on the edge of the tendon sheath during movement.

## Treatment

If the nodule is painless and does not affect the use of your hand, it is probably best left alone because it may settle by itself. If necessary, you can be given a steroid injection to shrink the nodule and free the tendon.

## Knee pain

Most people have painful knees at some time in their lives. In older people, osteoarthritis is common but there are many other causes of knee pain, especially in younger people. The knee is subjected to considerable stresses, especially if you are very overweight. Some sports, such as skiing and football, require your knees to rotate and bend and bear your weight at the same time, placing the knees under great strain.

All this means that the knees are susceptible to a wide range of injuries, often affecting the shock-absorbing cartilage pads within the joint and the many ligaments that hold the joint together (see diagram on page 68). Many injuries will heal naturally but some may need splints or even surgery.

## Pain under the heel

Pain in the sole of the foot, directly under the heel, is often caused by plantar fasciitis. This troublesome condition causes pain which is particularly severe when you first get out of bed in the morning but then eases a little as you continue to walk. The plantar fascia is a tough fibrous band, shaped like a triangle, which joins the ball of the foot with the heel bone. The strain and inflammation occur at the point where the fascia joins

## Anatomy of the knee

The bones of the knee are held together by strong ligaments.

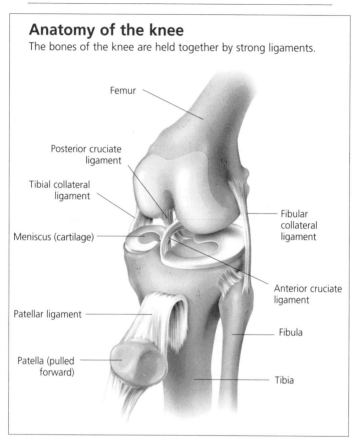

Femur

Posterior cruciate ligament

Tibial collateral ligament

Meniscus (cartilage)

Fibular collateral ligament

Anterior cruciate ligament

Patellar ligament

Fibula

Patella (pulled forward)

Tibia

the heel bone. Sometimes, an extra bit of bone, known as a spur, may grow at this point.

Plantar fasciitis often affects people who are on their feet a lot in their work and those who are overweight, so good footwear and losing weight can help. It can also be a feature of some types of inflammatory arthritis (see page 36), but this is unusual.

In older people, pain under the heel can also be the result of thinning of the fat pad. There is normally a

## Look after your knees

- Avoid squatting and kneeling, which strain the knees.

- Keep your weight down. If you are overweight, losing just a few pounds can help your pain and make all the difference to the strain on your knees.

- Avoid sitting in low, soft chairs. Getting out of them can be difficult if you have painful knees.

- Keep your thigh muscles strong with exercises (see page 94), especially if you play sports.

- Do not sleep with a pillow under your knees. It may feel comfortable but your knees can become permanently bent.

dense cushion of tissue, mostly fat, under the heel, which acts as a shock absorber when walking. This cushion may become thin as you get older and the heel bone is no longer so well protected. Well-fitting shoes with soft, sponge rubber soles and heels, perhaps with a soft insole as well, will protect the heels.

### Treatment
Steroid injection often helps plantar fasciitis but, because the injection can be very painful, other options may be tried first. These include an anti-inflammatory drug, wearing heel cups made of dense, shock-absorbing foam inside your shoes and strapping put on by a physiotherapist. Losing weight, if you are overweight, and avoiding prolonged standing can also help.

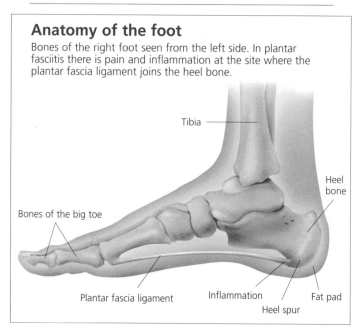

## Anatomy of the foot

Bones of the right foot seen from the left side. In plantar fasciitis there is pain and inflammation at the site where the plantar fascia ligament joins the heel bone.

Tibia

Heel bone

Bones of the big toe

Plantar fascia ligament

Inflammation

Heel spur

Fat pad

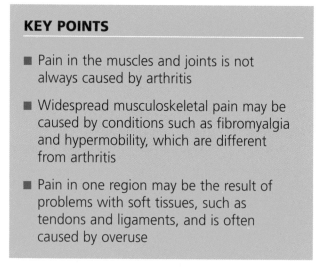

## KEY POINTS

- Pain in the muscles and joints is not always caused by arthritis

- Widespread musculoskeletal pain may be caused by conditions such as fibromyalgia and hypermobility, which are different from arthritis

- Pain in one region may be the result of problems with soft tissues, such as tendons and ligaments, and is often caused by overuse

# Treating arthritis and rheumatism

## A multidisciplined approach

Many people with locomotor problems will need more than one type of treatment – for example, drugs combined with physiotherapy and a programme of exercise to rehabilitate joints and soft tissues. Brief details of treatments for specific conditions are given in the preceding chapters. This section covers the treatments that may be used for arthritis and soft-tissue rheumatism in general.

## Drugs

Analgesics, or pain-killers, and non-steroidal anti-inflammatory drugs are the most important drugs in the treatment of arthritis and rheumatism. They are especially useful when the underlying cause of the symptoms cannot be cured.

## Analgesics

Examples of analgesics (often called 'simple analgesics' to distinguish them from anti-inflammatory drugs, which also act as pain-killers) are paracetamol, codeine, co-dydramol and dihydrocodeine. Paracetamol and codeine, and combinations of the two, are available over the counter under different trade names but the others are prescription-only drugs.

All of these medications, except paracetamol, can cause drowsiness and constipation. Co-proxamol is a simple analgesic which was widely used until recently. Now we know that it can be very dangerous in overdose, so it has been withdrawn.

Simple analgesics relieve pain but they do not have any anti-inflammatory action so they have little effect on stiffness and swelling.

## Anti-inflammatory drugs

Non-steroidal anti-inflammatory drugs (NSAIDs – pronounced 'en-seds') can often be very helpful when simple analgesics fail to relieve symptoms. They are so named because they reduce inflammation, which steroids also do, but they are completely different from steroids in the way that they work and in their potential side effects. NSAIDs are particularly effective in combating the stiffness and swelling that are caused by inflammation, as well as the pain.

The oldest anti-inflammatory drug is aspirin. Unfortunately, it needs to be given in large doses for it to have an anti-inflammatory effect (as distinct from a pain-killing effect) and in large doses it has a high risk of side effects, especially on the stomach. It has been superseded by more modern drugs with fewer side effects, such as ibuprofen, diclofenac and naproxen.

## Guidelines for using simple analgesics

- Start with paracetamol, which is the simplest, safest and cheapest analgesic, and which, if taken properly, is very effective.

- Always follow the instructions on the packaging and never exceed the recommended dose – all drugs are dangerous if you take too many, including paracetamol.

- If you have constant or frequent pain, take pain-killers regularly throughout the day, rather than waiting until the pain becomes really troublesome.

- If you have a lot of pain at night, take your pain-killers half an hour before bed-time.

- If you are planning a shopping trip or some other activity that you know will worsen your pain, take your pain-killers half an hour before you set off.

- If you find that the pain-killers that you are taking are not strong enough or you are taking them continuously, consult your doctor as there may be better pain-relieving strategies which could reduce your need for analgesics. Keep a record of how long each packet or bottle lasts you so that your doctor knows how many you've been taking.

**REMEMBER:** Many proprietary cold and flu treatments contain paracetamol, and there is a risk of an accidental overdose if you are already taking paracetamol regularly for pain relief.

## NSAIDs and the stomach

Why do NSAIDs cause stomach irritation? All NSAIDs work by blocking the production of prostaglandins in the tissues. Prostaglandins are chemicals released by cells at the site of an injury or damage caused by disease. They increase the flow of blood to the inflamed area, making it red and hot, and cause the blood vessels to become 'leaky', making the area swollen. Unfortunately, blocking prostaglandin production has negative as well as positive effects. This is because other types of prostaglandins, not involved in disease, play an important part in protecting the stomach lining from being damaged by its own digestive juices and acid. Unfortunately, NSAIDs block *all* prostaglandins, including the stomach protectors. This is why side effects such as indigestion, ulcers and bleeding from the stomach wall can all occur in people who take NSAIDs.

## COX-2 inhibitors

Newer NSAIDs (known as selective COX-2 or cyclo-oxygenase 2 inhibitors), such as celecoxib (Celebrex), etoricoxib (Arcoxia) and lumiracoxib (Prexige), appear to act in a specific way and their blocking effect is concentrated on the inflammatory prostaglandins rather than the protective ones (they reduce prostaglandin production at sites of pain and inflammation without affecting production in the stomach). In theory, these drugs look promising but it is not yet clear what their long-term side effects might be.

Several COX-2 inhibitors have been withdrawn because they have been associated with an increased risk of heart attacks and strokes.

As a result of these concerns, the Committee on Safety of Medicines advises that COX-2 inhibitors

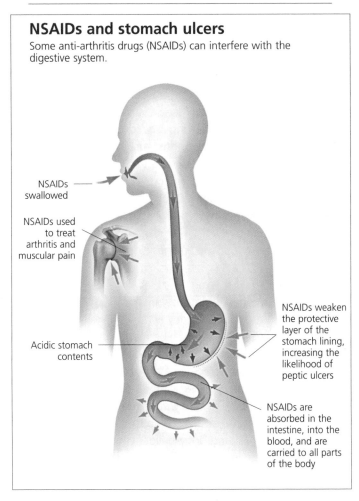

## NSAIDs and stomach ulcers

Some anti-arthritis drugs (NSAIDs) can interfere with the digestive system.

NSAIDs swallowed

NSAIDs used to treat arthritis and muscular pain

Acidic stomach contents

NSAIDs weaken the protective layer of the stomach lining, increasing the likelihood of peptic ulcers

NSAIDs are absorbed in the intestine, into the blood, and are carried to all parts of the body

should not be taken by people who have heart disease or vascular disease (diseases of blood vessels or 'hardening of the arteries').

However, it has become clear that COX-2 inhibitors have fewer gastrointestinal effects than NSAIDs, in particular the incidence of life-threatening ulcer complications such as bleeding and perforation.

At present this group of drugs is likely to be prescribed for you *only* if you develop gastric problems while on NSAIDs or have had ulcers in the past *and* if you do not have heart disease or vascular disease.

As a rule, NSAIDs offer most benefit to people with a form of inflammatory arthritis, such as rheumatoid arthritis, or who have developed an acute inflammation, such as gout. People with osteoarthritis and the soft-tissue problems described in the preceding chapter should begin with simple analgesics, which have fewer side effects, and change to an NSAID, for the shortest possible time, only if the analgesic does not work.

## Steroids

Steroids are produced naturally by the body. There are many different types and they act in many different ways. Many steroids can now be manufactured in the form of tablets and injections, and they are prescribed by doctors to treat a variety of conditions.

People often get worried when their doctor says that they need steroids. They have heard a lot about side effects and also about the abuse of steroids by certain sportsmen and body-builders. But the steroids used in arthritis are quite different from the ones abused in sports. The steroids used to treat arthritis are powerful anti-inflammatory drugs and they are very effective in controlling swelling, stiffness and pain. There is even some evidence from research that, in certain circumstances, they can reduce the damage done to joints by rheumatoid arthritis.

## Guidelines for using anti-inflammatory drugs (NSAIDs)

- Ibuprofen is the most widely available NSAID with the fewest side effects, so, unless your doctor advises otherwise, start with ibuprofen.

- Ibuprofen is available over the counter in a number of branded formulas but the unbranded or 'generic' version is cheaper and just as effective.

- If an NSAID reduces stiffness and swelling but you still have some pain, then also taking a simple analgesic, such as paracetamol, can be helpful. It is quite safe to do this as the two drugs work in different ways and do not interact.

- All NSAIDs must be taken with food and *never* on an empty stomach and, if you get a stomach upset, you must stop taking them. This is because they can irritate the lining of the stomach, causing indigestion and even ulcers and bleeding. All NSAIDs have this side effect to some extent, although only a minority of people who take them suffer from it.

- If you are elderly or if you have had an ulcer in the past, you are more susceptible to stomach irritation. You should consult your doctor before you take an NSAID. You may be given a combination treatment of an NSAID together with a drug to protect the stomach.

- If you have asthma, you need to be aware that occasionally aspirin and other NSAIDs may bring on an attack.

- Some NSAIDs are also available in the form of a gel that is massaged into the painful area. This can help pain that arises from the tissues near the surface of the skin, but is of little help in the pain of arthritis because the joints are too deep for the drug to penetrate to them.

Steroids can be taken in a variety of ways:

- In high doses for short periods to treat a flare in conditions such as systemic lupus erythematosus. The steroids may be given by mouth or, in severe cases, in hospital by direct injection into a vein.

- By single injection into the buttock muscle. This method is often used in people with rheumatoid arthritis who have just started taking drugs to control the arthritis long term. The steroid injection can tide them over while their drugs take effect – usually several weeks.

- In lower doses taken by mouth over the long term to keep inflammation under control in conditions such as polymyalgia rheumatica.

- Injected directly into a problem area such as an inflamed joint, tendon sheath or other soft tissue.

## Possible side effects of steroids

Like all drugs, steroids can have side effects. But despite the long list of side effects, steroids are powerful, effective drugs which are invaluable if used wisely (see 'Guidelines' on page 79). For example, when polymyalgia sufferers start taking steroids, they feel that they have been given a new lease of life.

## The possible side effects of long-term steroids

- Weight gain caused by an increase in appetite and retention of fluid.

- Raised blood pressure.

- Increased risk of developing diabetes and poor control of blood sugar levels in people who already have diabetes.

- Increased susceptibility to infections.

- Increased risk of stomach ulcers and bleeding.

- Increased risk of developing osteoporosis.

- Thinning of the skin and slow healing of cuts and grazes.

## Guidelines for taking long-term steroids

- Steroid treatment should always be prescribed and supervised by a doctor. Never adjust the dose except on the advice of a doctor.

- You will be given a blue card by the pharmacist when you start steroids. It carries the details of your steroid treatment and you should carry it with you at all times.

- If you are taken ill or injured, you must tell the doctor treating you that you take steroids and show him or her your blue card.

- Steroid tablets should be taken in the early morning, when the levels of natural steroids are at their peak. This causes less suppression of the adrenal glands.

- Instead of a dose every day, your doctor may suggest that you take double the dose on alternate days. This also can reduce the effect on the adrenal glands. Unfortunately, it is not always possible to do this as some people find that their symptoms are much worse on the non-steroid days.

- Once your condition has been controlled, if you need steroids long term, your doctor will reduce the dose to the lowest possible level to reduce the risk of side effects.

## Stopping steroids

When steroids are taken as treatment, they suppress the body's production of its own steroids, especially those made by the adrenal glands. These are small glands that sit on top of the kidneys and which produce steroids that control vital functions such as salt and water balance and blood pressure. If you stop taking steroids suddenly, you can become very ill because your adrenal glands need time to begin making their own steroids again. Therefore, steroids taken as treatment should always be tailed off gradually, to give the adrenal glands time to adjust.

## Steroid production in the adrenal glands

When steroids are taken as treatment, they suppress the body's production of its own steroids, especially those made by the adrenal glands.

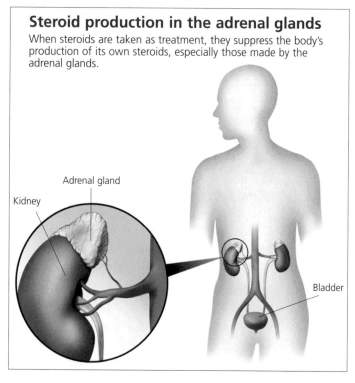

Adrenal gland

Kidney

Bladder

## Local steroid injections

If you have only one or two inflamed joints then steroids injected directly into the joints may be the best treatment. Many people with rheumatoid arthritis have repeated injections into their joints with great benefit. If the knee or the ankle is injected, it is safe to walk but you should rest the joint as much as possible for a day or two after the injection.

Steroid injections can also be given into painful and inflamed soft-tissue areas. This is a widely used and very effective form of treatment. Tennis elbow, tenosynovitis and carpal tunnel syndrome are often completely relieved by the injection of a small amount of steroid.

The injected steroid remains at the site of the injection and is slowly dispersed. Very little is absorbed into the rest of the body and so, in contrast to steroids taken by mouth, local steroid injections produce very few side effects. Occasionally, some people experience an increase in their pain for 24 hours but this settles as the steroid takes effect.

Local steroid injections carry a slight risk of wasting of the tissue and thinning of the skin at the injection site. This is seen as a small depression in the skin associated with loss of skin colour, which is more obvious in people with pigmented skin. The only disadvantage of this is cosmetic but for some people this is important so they should always be warned of the risk.

## Disease-modifying anti-rheumatoid drugs (DMARDs)

These are sulfasalazine, methotrexate, azathioprine, leflunomide (Arava), gold salts, penicillamine and hydroxychloroquine, and the newer drugs etanercept

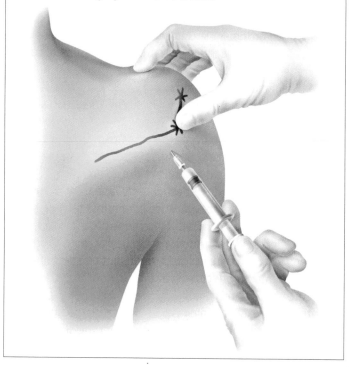

## A local injection of steroid

If you have only one or two inflamed joints then steroids injected directly into the joints may be the best answer. Here, the right shoulder is being injected from the back.

(Enbrel), infliximab (Remicade), adalimumab (Humira) and rituximab (MabThera).

They form a very important group of drugs but they are only ever used to treat widespread inflammatory arthritis, such as rheumatoid arthritis.

They are not used in other forms of arthritis and musculoskeletal conditions so information about them is included in the chapter on rheumatoid arthritis (see pages 21–9) rather than here.

## Antidepressant drugs

Some people with chronic, painful conditions may develop depression, making the pain even harder to cope with. There are several antidepressant drugs that help to lift the mood and ease the pain. Interestingly, certain types of pain, such as neuralgia, are eased by antidepressants even in people who are not depressed.

These very useful drugs are not addictive and, although some of the older drugs may cause drowsiness, newer ones do not.

## Physiotherapy

Many people with joint problems are referred to a physiotherapist for treatment. Physiotherapists are based in hospitals, some health centres and in private practices. Some are based in the community and can visit disabled people in their own homes. They are experts at maintaining the function of the locomotor system – that is, they will help you maintain strength and movement and reduce pain.

After a course of treatment, the physiotherapist may give you an exercise programme to do at home, to continue the benefit of your treatment. But physio- therapy cannot work miracles! It is important for you to keep your part of the bargain. Lose weight if you are overweight, perform your exercises regularly and take care to look after your joints.

## Hydrotherapy

Hydrotherapy is physiotherapy performed in a warm swimming pool. It is very effective at relieving the discomfort of stiff, painful joints. The water supports the weight of your body and the warmth helps your muscles relax and your joints to move. A course of hydrotherapy can give prolonged benefit in conditions such as osteoarthritis of the hip and ankylosing spondylitis.

## Surgery

Many people with arthritis assume that the only thing a surgeon can do to help is to replace a damaged joint. This is probably the most common operation, but it is by no means the only form of surgical treatment available.

Your doctor may discuss the possibility of surgery with you if one or more joints have become so damaged, painful and stiff that you can no longer use them properly, despite taking pain-killers and regular exercise.

### Surgical options
#### Arthroscopy

This is a form of 'keyhole' surgery usually performed under a general anaesthetic, but as a day case (that is, the patient is discharged from the hospital after the procedure, on the same day). It is used to diagnose and treat problems within a joint, most often injury to the knee. A thin tube passed through a small incision in the skin allows the surgeon to see into the joint. Other surgical instruments inserted through further small incisions allow the surgeon to perform small operations.

#### Synovectomy

This operation removes inflamed synovium from within joints and around tendons in people with rheumatoid arthritis. Although it can help to relieve symptoms and may slow the progress of the disease, it is not a cure and the inflamed tissue often re-forms, sometimes quite quickly. For this reason, it is always used together with drug treatment.

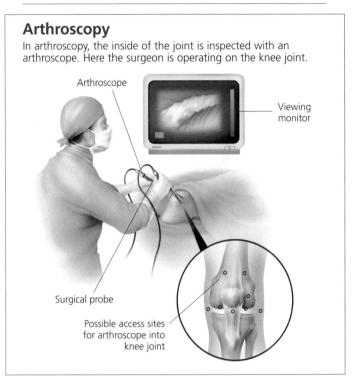

## Arthroscopy

In arthroscopy, the inside of the joint is inspected with an arthroscope. Here the surgeon is operating on the knee joint.

Arthroscope

Viewing monitor

Surgical probe

Possible access sites
for arthroscope into
knee joint

### Tendon and ligament surgery

Surgery can be performed to realign tendons or loosen tight tendon sheaths and even, in some cases, to repair broken tendons.

### Osteotomy

If one area of a joint surface is badly damaged but other parts are still in a relatively good condition, surgery to realign the bone may redirect the pressure away from the damaged area. Osteotomy is sometimes used in younger people with arthritis to postpone the need for joint replacement.

## Osteotomy

An osteotomy creates a surgical fracture – in this case so that the hip may be realigned when the bone is rejoined.

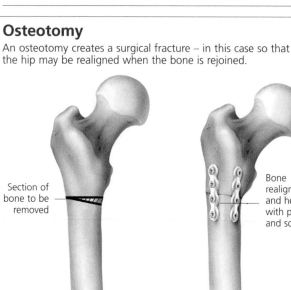

Section of bone to be removed

Bone realigned and held with plates and screws

### Arthrodesis

This is surgery to fuse a joint so that it can no longer move. It abolishes pain but the joint is left completely stiff. It is a very useful operation for severe arthritis affecting the feet, ankles, wrists and occasionally in the spine.

### Arthroplasty or joint replacement

Artificial joints for hips and knees have been widely used for over 30 years and have a very high success rate. In certain cases, shoulders, elbows and finger joints can be replaced, although the surgery is technically more difficult. For more information on joint replacement, see the book *Understanding Hip and Knee Arthritis Surgery* in the Family Doctor series.

## Arthrodesis

Arthrodesis means fusion of a joint to eliminate joint pain. Here the heel bone has been joined to a bone in the centre of the foot using a metal plate.

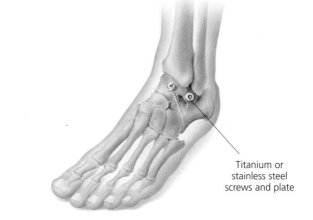

Titanium or stainless steel screws and plate

### Hip replacement

The two parts of a hip replacement are the metal femoral component (artificial upper thigh bone) and the plastic acetabular component (artificial hip socket). The combination of metal and plastic is very hard wearing.

### Knee replacement

The two parts of a knee replacement are the femoral component and the tibial component. Again, a combination of metal and plastic is used.

## Complementary medicine

Many people who have arthritis or rheumatism feel that they gain benefit from complementary medicines and use them as well as their conventional medicines. This may be because orthodox treatment is unable to control their symptoms completely and also because

## Hip replacement

The two parts of a hip replacement are the femoral component (artificial upper thigh bone) and the acetabular component (artificial hip socket).

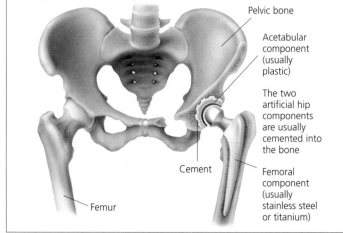

Pelvic bone

Acetabular component (usually plastic)

The two artificial hip components are usually cemented into the bone

Cement

Femoral component (usually stainless steel or titanium)

Femur

## Knee replacement

A knee replacement comprises two or three components: a metal femoral component, a plastic tibial component and a plastic replacement patella.

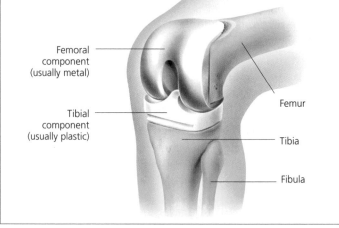

Femoral component (usually metal)

Tibial component (usually plastic)

Femur

Tibia

Fibula

they believe that complementary therapies are natural and safer.

Although there is some truth in this view, it is not the whole story and there are other factors that you should bear in mind before deciding whether to try the complementary approach (see box on page 90).

In fact, it can be very difficult to make an objective assessment as to whether complementary methods and treatments are effective. Few have been scientifically tested, so there is little reliable evidence as to whether they actually work. The picture is complicated by the fact that the symptoms of arthritis may vary over time regardless of treatment, making it difficult to judge whether an improvement is the result of a particular treatment or simply part of the normal pattern of the disease.

Although many types of therapy are safe, you cannot always assume that this is so. In particular, you should be wary of herbal remedies imported from abroad and distributed by small-scale practitioners or shops. The quality of these products is not controlled and, in the past, some have been found to contain powerful drugs such as steroids or even poisonous heavy metals.

## Copper bracelets
These are a traditional remedy for all kinds of aches and pains, but there is no real evidence that they are effective. However, they are unlikely to be harmful.

## Glucosamine and chondroitin sulphate
These dietary supplements contain substances found naturally in the body which play a role in strength-ening cartilage and help it to retain water. Some

## Using complementary medicines

- Do as much research as you can into the training and experience of the therapist. Reputable ones are likely to be registered with a regulatory body that monitors practitioners. Be especially wary of anyone who promises you a cure.

- Tell your doctor if you are using other types of treatment. Occasionally there may be undesirable interactions between conventional and complementary medicines.

- As with any medicine, always read the instructions on the pack and do not exceed the recommended dose. It can be tempting to assume that 'more is better', but this is unlikely to be the case.

- Never stop taking conventional treatments without consulting your doctor, especially if you are taking steroids, as stopping them suddenly can be dangerous.

- Try to relate the cost of treatment to its effectiveness – if you see no improvement after a reasonable time, there is no point in wasting your money. One way of doing this is to keep a diary of your symptoms for a month or so before starting any complementary treatment, and continue for another month once you are using it. You can then use this information to see whether you feel that the therapy is making any difference.

research has suggested that taking supplements may encourage damaged cartilage to repair itself, and even prevent cartilage damage in the first place, without causing side effects. Other research has shown no benefit. Some people find that the supplements help their pain but the ideal dose and formulation have not been identified, nor is it clear whether the effects will be long lasting.

The NICE (National Institute for Health and Clinical Excellence) is the organisation that assesses drugs and treatments for the National Health Service, and it does not recommend glucosamine and chondroitin sulphate as effective treatments.

## Fish oils

Fish oils and evening primrose oil contain essential fatty acids (called 'essential' because the body cannot make them but must obtain them from food). There is now good scientific evidence that these oils can reduce inflammation in arthritis, although the effect is small. Cod liver oil contains essential fatty acids, together with vitamin D, which helps to absorb calcium. However, it also contains vitamin A and so should not be taken in large amounts as excess vitamin A can be dangerous.

## Acupuncture

This traditional Chinese therapy involves inserting fine needles into the skin at certain carefully defined points to liberate the flow of 'ki', sometimes called the 'life force'. Modern research suggests that it may help to reduce pain by stimulating the body to produce natural pain-killing chemicals called 'endorphins'. In China, acupuncture is used to treat a wide range of medical conditions and even to provide anaesthesia for surgical operations.

In the west, there is some scientific evidence that it helps certain types of musculoskeletal pain and many physiotherapy departments now use it in a limited way. If you consult a private practitioner, make sure that he or she is registered. In skilled hands, the procedure is very safe.

## Homoeopathy

Homoeopathy was devised as a system of medicine in the late nineteenth century and homoeopathic remedies are widely used today. The principle of treatment is that 'like cures like': in other words, a homoeopath will choose remedies that, in larger amounts, would cause the symptoms being treated.

The actual choice of remedies will be based on your answers to extensive questioning about your history, symptoms and personality. The remedies are made from substances extracted from plants, minerals and animals, diluted many times.

Homoeopaths hold that, as the substances are diluted, they become more 'potent' and high-potency preparations are so dilute that they probably do not contain a single molecule of the original substance. Side effects and drug interactions are rare.

## Osteopathy, chiropractic and Alexander technique

These are therapies with some similarities to physiotherapy, although they developed in very different ways. They are not usually available under the National Health Service but are widely available privately. They can be particularly effective for spinal problems.

Alexander technique can be helpful in correcting faulty posture. Practitioners teach how to use the body correctly and inhibit ingrained habits of poor posture and incorrect movement. Breathing techniques are also taught to aid movement.

Chiropractic is a variant of osteopathy. The two therapies are very similar and deal with biomechanical problems. They see pain and disability as arising from flaws in the function of the locomotor system. These flaws need not cause symptoms but may throw excessive strain on other parts of the locomotor system.

## KEY POINTS

- Many different types of drug are useful in the treatment of locomotor problems

- Some people avoid drugs that could help them considerably because of misplaced fears – do not be afraid to take the drugs that your doctor recommends but, if you have concerns, do talk to your doctor about them

- Complementary medicines and therapies can help the symptoms of arthritis and rheumatism

- There is usually little scientific evidence that complementary medicines or therapies have a fundamental effect on diseases so, if they do not help your symptoms, they are best abandoned

- Always consult registered complementary practitioners and buy medicines from reputable shops and pharmacies

# Living with arthritis and rheumatism

## Exercise

Many people believe that they should rest their arthritic joints and that this will prevent further damage. In fact, the right kind of exercise is not only beneficial but *essential* for keeping the joints mobile and the muscles strong. Prolonged rest, on the other hand, usually leads to more stiffness and to weakness and wasting of the muscles, while having no effect on the pain.

Nevertheless, the wrong kind of exercise is worse than none at all. For example, touching your toes and 'sit-ups' put an enormous strain on the lumbar region of the spine.

You should also avoid 'the squat' – bending your knees and hips from a standing position until your bottom touches your heels then standing up again. This exercise really punishes your knees.

Do not rotate your head round like a windmill, hoping that this is a good exercise for your neck, because it can actually cause strain.

And lastly, never crack the joints in your fingers. What begins as a party trick can become a habit and can, over time, damage the joints.

Aim to include three types of exercise in your programme:

- stretching exercises

- muscle-strengthening exercises

- general fitness or aerobic exercises.

The programme will also include a 'weight-bearing' element to help strengthen your bones and reduce your risk of developing osteoporosis. A good exercise programme should be part of your daily routine, whether or not you have arthritis.

## Your exercise programme

Always start with gentle exercises and then build up gradually. The right sort of exercise should not cause pain, so listen to your body and adjust your activities accordingly.

### Stretching

Stretching involves putting each of your joints through a full range of movement every day. Begin at the top of your body and work downwards so that no area is forgotten.

#### Neck

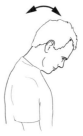

- Drop your head forwards on to your chest and let it hang there for a few seconds.

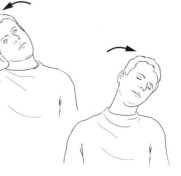

- Then straighten up and drop your head to the side, again letting it hang for a few seconds. Repeat, dropping your head to the other side.

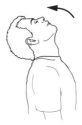

- Turn round to look over your shoulder as far as you can and hold the position for a few seconds. Repeat, turning to the other side.

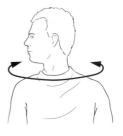

- Tip your head back as far as you can but do not force it, and this time do not hold the position for more than a second because you may feel dizzy.

### Shoulders

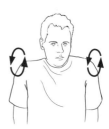

With your arms by your sides, rotate your shoulders in circles a few times, first forwards and then backwards.

- Lift your arms up above your head, bringing them in against your ears and pushing them backwards at the same time. Hold the position for a few seconds and then slowly bring them down sideways.

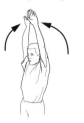

- Put your hands behind your back and clasp them. Then push your clasped hands backwards, away from your trunk and hold for a few seconds.

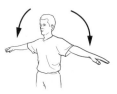

### Elbows

- Straighten your elbows and then bend them up as far as they will go.

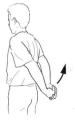

- Then, with your arms tucked into your sides and your elbows bent to 90 degrees, turn your forearms so that your palms are facing upwards and then downwards.

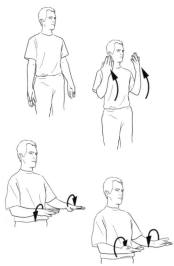

## Wrists and hands

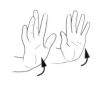

- Bend your wrists up and down as far as they will go.

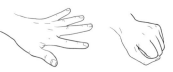

- Spread your fingers out hard and then clench your fists. Do this several times. If your fingers do not straighten fully, put your hand on a flat surface palm downwards and very gently push the bent joints down with your other hand. Similarly, if your fingers do not close fully into a fist, very gently push them down with your other hand.

- Bring your thumb and index finger together in a pinch and then touch the tips of your other fingers in turn with your thumb. Repeat with your other hand.

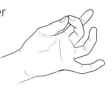

- The muscles in your hands can be strengthened by repeatedly squashing a soft rubber ball into your palm, allowing it to inflate fully between squashes.

## Upper back (thoracic spine)

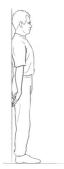

- Stand with your back against a wall and straighten your back so that the back of your head touches the wall. Hold for a few seconds.

- Sit down and twist your trunk and shoulders round to one side as far as you can, hold for a few seconds and repeat to the other side.

- Take a deep breath in, expanding your chest as much as possible and hold for a few seconds.

## Lower back (lumbar spine)

- Stand up straight and lean over to one side, running your hand down the side of your leg. Do not force the movement but just hang there for a few seconds. Repeat on the other side.

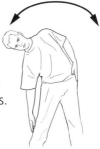

- Lie flat on the floor with your knees bent up. Lift your pelvis off the floor by tightening your stomach muscles and hold for a few seconds.

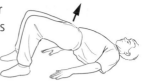

- Now straighten your legs out in front of you and push the small of your back against the floor, holding for a few seconds.

- Kneel on the floor on all fours. Make an arch of your back and then a hollow. Repeat several times (this exercise is known as 'the cat').

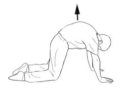

### Hips

- Sit on the floor with your legs out in front of you and separate them out to the sides as far as they will go and hold for a few seconds.

- Then bring your legs together and bend your knees up to your chest, one at a time if this is more comfortable. Hug your knees to your chest with your arms and hold them there for a few seconds (this is also a good exercise for your knees).

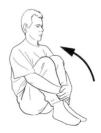

- Stand up and hold on to a chair back or table for support. Lift one leg and swing it back behind you as far as it will go. Repeat with the other leg.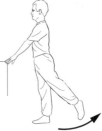

### Knees

- Sit on a bed or on the floor with your back supported and your legs straight out in front of you. Push the backs of your knees hard against the surface, feeling the big quadriceps muscle in the front of your thigh tighten as you do so, and hold for a few seconds.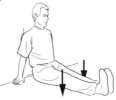

- Lift one leg up, keeping the knee straight, until your heel is about six inches above the surface. Once again, feel the quadriceps muscle working and hold for a few seconds. Repeat with the other leg.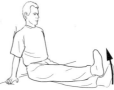

- Find a low step and step on and off, alternating with each leg.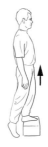

## Ankles and feet

- Rotate your ankles in circles, first clockwise and then anti-clockwise.

- Bend your ankles up to bring your toes towards you and then bend them away from you, pointing your toes like a ballet dancer.

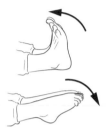

- Wiggle your toes.

## Strengthening

Strengthening exercises work the muscles harder. Strong muscles are very important in helping to protect the joints from strain. Many of the exercises above will strengthen your muscles as well as stretching your joints.

More advanced muscle-strengthening exercises make the muscles work harder by lifting weights. The weights should be carefully chosen to suit you personally or the group of muscles being worked so try to get advice from a qualified person such as a physiotherapist or gym trainer. Weights that cause pain are too heavy.

## Aerobic

Aerobic exercise works your heart and lungs as well as some of your joints and increases your stamina. Activities such as swimming, brisk walking and using an exercise bicycle are good examples. An exercise bicycle is particularly beneficial if you have arthritis in your hips or knees as the bicycle exercises these joints without them having to carry your weight at the same time. Swimming is a good choice if you are overweight because, again, the joints are exercised without having to support your body weight.

A moderate amount of exercise performed regularly, say two or three times a week, is much better for you than a blitz once a month, or only when you feel guilty. And even a small amount of exercise done regularly, such as a daily 10-minute walk, is much better than doing nothing.

## Protecting your joints

Besides regular exercise, looking after your joints also involves protecting them from unnecessary strain in your everyday activities. People with arthritis can avoid pain and preserve their independence by making changes in the way that they do things. This is not 'giving in to arthritis' but simply good sense. Occupational therapists are experts in helping people to function as normally as possible, and advising on joint protection is one aspect of their work. They are based in hospitals and in social services departments and, if necessary, they will visit you at home to advise on aids, appliances and adaptations. Aids for every aspect of daily living are displayed in showrooms run by the Disabled Living Foundation (see Useful addresses, page 117).

People with healthy joints can also benefit from simple advice on joint protection. Avoiding unnecessary strain makes good sense for them too. It can make difficult or tiring tasks easier and it can help to avoid problems in the future. An obvious place to start easing the strain is in the kitchen (see box below).

It is much easier on the hips and knees to get up from a high-seated chair with arms and out of a bath with handles. Shoes with soft, rubber cushion soles act as shock absorbers and can protect the joints while walking. A walking stick can also be enormously helpful.

## Walking with a stick

If you have problems with your knees or hips, a walking stick can make a huge difference to your comfort, confidence and mobility. A walking stick, when used correctly, can take the load off an arthritic joint and help protect it from strain.

### Tips in the kitchen

- A perching stool takes the weight off your legs when you are working at the sink, work-surface or ironing board.

- Steam irons are heavy and should be avoided if you have wrist, elbow or shoulder problems.

- Saucepans with two handles share the load between both hands.

- Eye-level shelves and cupboards are less tiring than floor cupboards, as reaching up causes less strain than bending.

You can buy these walking sticks in chemists and elsewhere but there are many different types. It is best to get expert advice on the right one from a physio-therapist or occupational therapist who can assess your needs and help you to make the right choice.

## Arthritis and the weather

At the first sign of cool, damp weather in the autumn, many people with arthritis and rheumatism find that their symptoms get worse. On the other hand, during the summer months or when they are on holiday, their arthritis is much less troublesome. Sometimes it can seem as if your joints are acting as a barometer. Although this experience is very common, we do not know why joint pain and stiffness are so sensitive to changes in the weather. But we do know that adverse weather conditions do not cause arthritis and they do not make existing arthritis worse.

Although people living in warm climates complain less of joint pain and stiffness, they develop the same forms of arthritis and often show abnormalities on their X-rays similar to those of people living in cool climates. Warmth is soothing and aids muscle relaxation and this is undoubtedly important in easing symptoms.

In warm weather and especially on holiday, people are often more active and the exercise is also beneficial to stiff, painful joints.

If you have arthritis, you should keep warm and try to maintain your levels of activity even when the weather is cold. A warm bath followed by a simple programme of exercises can help enormously to reduce the pain and stiffness of arthritic joints.

## Diet and arthritis

People often wonder if their diet has anything to do with their arthritis. The answer is, 'probably not'! The one exception is gout (discussed on pages 30–5), where alcohol and foods containing large amounts of purines, such as liver, heart, kidney and fish roe, can make the condition worse. Food allergies as a cause of arthritis are highly individual, difficult to test for and probably very rare. However, if you feel that a certain food makes your symptoms worse, then you can do an experiment called an 'exclusion diet' to test this out (see box below).

There are lots of published 'diets for arthritis', supported by glowing testimonials from people who claim that their particular diet 'cured' their arthritis and

### Exclusion diet

- Keep a diary of your joint pain and stiffness for six weeks.

- For the first two weeks, eat a normal diet, including the suspect food.

- For the second two weeks, cut the suspect food out of your diet completely.

- For the third two weeks, include the suspect food in your diet again.

- If your symptoms improve during the middle two weeks when you exclude the food, and then get worse again when you reintroduce it during the last two weeks, then it is reasonable to conclude that the suspect food is making your symptoms worse.

will cure yours too! Unfortunately, glowing testimonials do not amount to scientific evidence and you may waste a lot of money following a diet that has no good evidence to support it.

The best diet for arthritis is a healthy diet – one with a balance of protein, carbohydrate and fat with plenty of fibre, vitamins, calcium, iron and other minerals. A good diet will also help you to keep close to your ideal weight – and keeping your weight down is one of the most important things that you can do to take the strain off your joints.

## Arthritis and inheritance

Many people with arthritis want to know if the arthritis will 'run in the family'. It is certainly true that almost all forms have an inherited element – that is, if you have arthritis then your first-degree relatives (children and siblings) have an increased chance of developing it too. But for most forms of arthritis, the increased risk is still very small indeed. And even if they do develop arthritis, it may still be mild, even if your arthritis is one of the severe forms. We cannot predict ahead of time who will and who won't develop arthritis and, more importantly, we cannot prevent it. The best advice is to lead a healthy life, take regular exercise, don't abuse your joints and don't worry. Whatever form of arthritis you have, the chance that your child or grandchild will also have arthritis is very small.

## Pain control

Pain should always be respected and constantly pushing yourself to continue activities that make it worse is counterproductive. On the other hand, too little activity is as bad as too much because it can leave

# What should you weigh?

- The body mass index (BMI) is a useful measure of healthy weight
- Find out your height in metres and weight in kilograms
- Calculate your BMI like this:

$$BMI = \frac{\text{Your weight (kg)}}{[\text{Your height (metres)} \times \text{Your height (metres)}]}$$

$$\text{e.g. } 24.8 = \frac{70}{[1.68 \times 1.68]}$$

- You are recommended to try to maintain a BMI in the range 18.5–24.9
- The chart below is an easier way of estimating your BMI. Read off your height and your weight. The point where the lines cross in the chart indicates your BMI

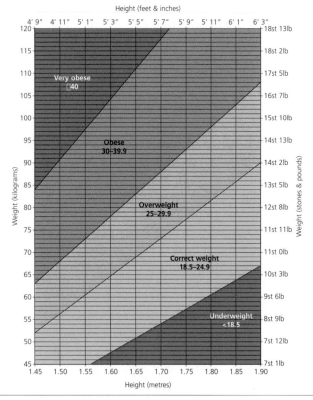

you with weakened muscles and encourage joints to stiffen and lose flexibility. There are many techniques for reducing pain besides drugs, and some of them you can easily try for yourself at home (see box on page 110).

## The future

There are over 200 types of arthritis and, for many types, there is no single cause. Therefore, a single 'cure for arthritis' is very unlikely to be found! But for people with arthritis of all kinds, there is a great deal of help available and even people with severe arthritis can remain mobile and independent. In fact, most people with arthritis can lead normal lives.

On the other side of the coin is the fact that the population is living longer and people of all ages complain more about pain, stiffness and other locomotor problems. What is the cause of this? Certainly, it does not seem that the more serious forms of arthritis, such as rheumatoid arthritis, are becoming more common. Some of this increased stiffness, disability and pain is undoubtedly caused by osteoarthritis, which is more common in people who are older. But much is also the result of body abuse – lack of exercise, overweight, poor posture and overuse syndromes are the scourges of modern life in affluent societies. Abolishing these scourges would reduce not only locomotor problems but also diabetes, high blood pressure and heart disease.

The remedy is largely in our own hands. You will notice how much I have emphasised the importance of exercise throughout this book. Exercise, exercise and exercise are probably the three most important factors in keeping the joints healthy! Daily working lives are

## Practical pain control

**Ice packs:** you can buy cold packs to keep in the home freezer and use when you need them. If you use a bag of ice or a pack of frozen peas instead, wrap it in a tea towel to protect your skin and apply it for no longer than 20 minutes. Cold packs are helpful for acute inflammation and swelling but avoid them if you have poor circulation or skin numbness.

**Hot packs:** these may be electric or ones that you heat yourself (including microwaveable types) and are used in the same way as cold packs. Heat lamps work in a similar way, and don't neglect the traditional hot bath as a form of pain relief. Heat is good if you have deep aching pain, especially with muscle tension. Again, you shouldn't use hot packs if you have poor circulation or skin numbness because of the danger of accidental burns.

**TENS (transcutaneous electrical nerve stimulation):** this method of pain relief uses simple equipment to deliver a mild electric current through pads attached to the skin over painful areas. Stimulating nerves in this way blocks the pain sensations and prevents them reaching the brain. The equipment is safe and easy to use and is often especially helpful for hip, shoulder and back pain. If you would like to try TENS then ask your physiotherapist.

**Massage:** if you have a partner, friend or relative who is willing to learn how to give you a simple oil massage, this traditional form of therapy can be a big help in relieving pain, especially in the muscles. Either ask an expert to demonstrate or buy one of the many excellent books on the topic.

now much less active compared with 50 years ago.
On the other hand, exercise classes, swimming pools
and gyms for leisure time are now widely available,
with activities to suit almost everyone of whatever age.
Find out about them today!

## KEY POINTS

- The right sort of exercise, performed
  regularly, is essential for keeping your
  locomotor system in the best possible
  condition

- The ideal is a balance of stretching for
  your joints, strengthening for your
  muscles and aerobic exercise for stamina

# Useful addresses

We have included the following organisations because, on preliminary investigation, they may be of use to the reader. However, we do not have first-hand experience of each organisation and so cannot guarantee the organisation's integrity. The reader must therefore exercise his or her own discretion and judgement when making further enquiries.

**Arthritis and Musculoskeletal Alliance (ARMA)**
Bride House, 18–20 Bride Lane
London EC4Y 8EE
Tel: 020 7842 0910
Website: www.arma.uk.net

Brings together support groups, professional bodies and research organisations in the field of arthritis and other musculoskeletal conditions.

**Arthritis Care**
18 Stephenson Way
London NW1 2HD

Te: 020 7380 6500
Helpline: 0808 800 4050
Website: www.arthritiscare.org.uk

Provides information, counselling, training and social contact. The first port of call for anyone with arthritis, including gout. Many smaller organisations for particular types of arthritis; for details ring helpline or freephone.

**Arthritis Research Campaign**
Copeman House, St Mary's Court, St Mary's Gate
Chesterfield, Derbyshire S41 7TD
Tel: 0870 850 5000
Website: www.arc.org.uk

Finances an extensive programme of research and education in a wide range of arthritis and rheumatism problems including back pain. Provides useful booklets explaining related problems and ways of coping with them.

**Assist UK (Disabled Living Centres Council)**
Redbank House, 4 St Chad's Street
Manchester M8 8QA
Tel: 0870 770 2866
Textphone: 0870 770 5813
Website: www.assist-uk.org

Leads a network of over 50 local centres throughout the UK where furniture, appliances, aids and adaptations for disabled and elderly people are displayed. Has a wide range of services for clients, manufacturers and statutory sector. Offers training courses for health professionals. Information leaflets available on request.

**BackCare (The Charity for Healthier Backs)**
16 Elmtree Road
Teddington, Middlesex TW11 8ST
Tel: 020 8977 5474
Helpline: 0845 130 2704
Website: www.backcare.org.uk

Offers information and advice for people with back
pain. Funds patient-oriented scientific research into
the causes, treatment and prevention of back pain.
Has local support groups throughout the country with
regular meetings.

**Benefits Enquiry Line**
Tel: 0800 882200
Minicom: 0800 243355
Website: www.dwp.gov.uk
N. Ireland: 0800 220674

Government agency giving information and advice on
sickness and disability benefits for people with
disabilities and their carers.

**British Acupuncture Council**
63 Jeddo Road
London W12 9HQ
Tel: 020 8735 0400 (Mon–Fri 9.30am–5.30pm)
Website: www.acupuncture.org.uk

Professional body offering information about the
therapy and lists of qualified acupuncture therapists.

**British Association of Occupational Therapists and College of Occupational Therapists**
106–114 Borough High Street
London SE1 1LB
Tel: 020 7357 6480
Website: www.cot.org.uk

For information about all aspects of occupational therapy. An SAE requested.

**British Homeopathic Association**
Hahnemann House, 29 Park Street West
Luton LU1 3BE
Tel: 01582 408675
Website: www.trusthomeopathy.org

Professional body representing qualified homoeopathic practitioners. Offers information about homoeopathy, research, hospitals and clinics providing homoeopathy under the NHS, as well as lists of private practitioners.

**CCAA (Children's Chronic Arthritis Association)**
Ground Floor, Amber Gate, City Wall Road
Worcester WR1 2AH
Tel: 01905 745595
Website: www.ccaa.org.uk

Offers information and practical support to families of children with juvenile idiopathic arthritis. Arranges educational and recreational opportunities for children with arthritis.

**Chartered Society of Physiotherapy**
14 Bedford Row
London WC1R 4ED
Tel: 020 7306 6666
Website: www.csp.org.uk

For information about all aspects of physiotherapy.
Offers lists of registered physiotherapists around the
country.

**Clinical Knowledge Summaries**
Sowerby Centre for Health Informatics at Newcastle
(SCHIN Ltd), Bede House, All Saints Business Centre
Newcastle upon Tyne NE1 2ES
Tel: 0191 243 6100
Website: www.cks.library.nhs.uk

A website mainly for GPs giving information for
patients listed by disease plus named self-help
organisations.

**Contact a Family**
209–211 City Road
London EC1V 1JN
Textphone: 0808 808 3556
Helpline: 0808 808 3555 (Mon–Fri 10am–4pm,
Mon 5.30–7.30pm)
Website: www.cafamily.org.uk

Has information on over 1,000 rare disorders and
disabilities and can put families in touch with each
other for mutual support.

**Crossroads Association**
10 Regent Place
Rugby, Warwickshire CV21 2PN
Tel: 0845 450 0350
Website: www.crossroads.org.uk

Provides reliable, fully trained care support workers free to give the regular carers of ill or frail people 'time to be themselves'.

**Disabled Living Foundation**
380–384 Harrow Road
London W9 2HU
Helpline: 0845 130 9177 (Mon–Fri 10am–4pm)
Tel: 020 7289 6111 (Mon–Fri 9am–5pm)
Textphone 020 7432 8009
Website: www.dlf.org.uk

Provides information to disabled and elderly people on all kinds of equipment in order to promote their independence and quality of life.

**Fibromyalgia Association UK**
PO Box 206, Stourbridge
West Midlands DY9 8YL
Helpline: 0845 345 2322 (Mon–Fri 10am–4pm)
Benefits helpline: 0845 345 2343 (Mon, Fri 10am–12 noon)
Website: www.fibromyalgia-associationuk.org

Provides information for patients with fibromyalgia and has a network of local support groups throughout the UK. Campaigns for a better recognition and awareness of the disorder.

**General Osteopathic Council**
Osteopathy House, 176 Tower Bridge Road
London SE1 3LU
Tel: 020 7357 6655
Website: www.osteopathy.org.uk

Regulatory body that offers information to the public
and lists of accredited osteopaths.

**Hypermobility Syndrome Association**
49 Orchard Crescent, Oreston
Plymouth PL9 7NF
Tel: 0845 345 4465
Website: www.hypermobility.org.uk

Charity run by and for people with hypermobility
syndrome. For information please send an SAE.

**mobilise**
**(Promoting mobility for disabled people)**
National Headquarters, Ashwellthorpe
Norwich NR16 1EX
Tel: 01508 489449
Website: www.mobilise.info

Self-help association offering information and advice,
and campaigning for independence through mobility
with a wide range of services.

**National Ankylosing Spondylitis Society (NASS)**
Unit 0.2, 1 Victoria Villas
Richmond, Surrey TW9 2GW
Tel: 020 8948 9117
Website: www.nass.co.uk

Provides information and advice to patients with ankylosing spondylitis, their families and professionals. Has over 100 branches providing supervised physiotherapy one evening a week. Videos, cassette tapes and DVDs of physiotherapy exercises available.

## National Institute for Health and Clinical Excellence (NICE)

MidCity Place, 71 High Holborn
London WC1V 6NA
Tel: 0845 003 7780
Website: www.nice.org.uk

Provides national guidance on the promotion of good health and the prevention and treatment of ill-health. Patient information leaflets are available for each piece of guidance issued.

## National Osteoporosis Society

Manor Farm, Skinners Hill, Camerton
Bath, Somerset BA2 0PJ
Tel: 0845 130 3076/01761 471771 (Mon–Thurs, 9am–4.30pm, Fri 9am–4pm)
Helpline: 0845 450 0230 (Mon–Fri 9am–5pm)
Website: www.nos.org.uk

Provides information, advice on all aspects of osteoporosis, the menopause and hormone replacement therapy. Encourages people to take action to protect their bones. Helpline staffed by specially trained nurses. Has local support groups.

**National Rheumatoid Arthritis Society**
Unit B4, Westacott Business Centre
Westacott Way, Littlewick Green, Maidenhead SL6 3RT
Tel: 0845 458 3969
Helpline: 0800 298 7650
Website: www.rheumatoid.org.uk

Provides information, education and support for people
with rheumatoid arthritis, their families and carers.

**NHS Direct**
Tel: 0845 4647 (24 hours, 365 days a year)
Website: www.nhsdirect.nhs.uk

Offers confidential health-care advice, information and
referral service. A good first port of call for any health
advice.

**NHS Smoking Helpline**
Freephone: 0800 022 4332 (7am–11pm, 365 days a
year)
Website: http://smokefree.nhs.uk
Pregnancy smoking helpline: 0800 169 9169
(12 noon–9pm, 365 days a year)

Have advice, help and encouragement on giving up
smoking. Specialist advisers available to offer ongoing
support to those who genuinely are trying to give up
smoking. Can refer to local branches.

**Patients' Association**
PO Box 935
Harrow, Middlesex HA1 3YJ
Tel: 020 8423 9111

Helpline: 0845 608 4455
Website: www.patients-association.com

Provides advice on patients' rights, leaflets and a directory of self-help groups.

**Quit (Smoking Quitlines)**
63 St Mary's Axe
London EC3 8AA
Helpline: 0800 002200 (9am–9pm, 365 days a year)
Tel: 020 7469 0400
Website: www.quit.org.uk

Offers individual advice on giving up smoking in English and Asian languages. Talks to schools on smoking and pregnancy and can refer to local support groups. Runs training courses for professionals.

**RADAR**
12 City Forum, 250 City Road
London EC1V 8AF
Tel: 020 7250 3222
Minicom: 020 7250 4119
Website: www.radar.org.uk

Campaigning body run by and for disabled people. Sells key to access locked public lavatories for £3.50.

**Society of Teachers of the Alexander Technique (STAT)**
1st Floor, Linton House, 39–51 Highgate Road
London NW5 1RS
Tel: 020 7482 5135
Website: www.stat.org.uk

Offers general information and lists of teachers of the Alexander Technique in the UK and worldwide and recommended training schools. Members receive up-to-date information.

## Useful websites
### BBC
**www.bbc.co.uk/health**
A helpful website: easy to navigate and offers lots of useful advice and information. Also contains links to other related topics.

### Bodytalkonline
**www.bodytalk-online.com**
Series of online presentations about different medical conditions.

### Care directions
**www.carersinformation.org.uk**
Resource for supporting informal carers.

### Healthtalkonline
**www.healthtalkonline.org**
Website of the DIPEx charity.

### NHS choices
**www.nhs.uk/conditions**
Government's patient information portal.

### Patient UK
**www.patient.co.uk**
Patient care website.

## The internet as a source of further information

After reading this book, you may feel that you would like further information on the subject. The internet is of course an excellent place to look and there are many websites with useful information about medical disorders, related charities and support groups.

For those who do not have a computer at home some bars and cafes offer facilities for accessing the internet. These are listed in the *Yellow Pages* under 'Internet Bars and Cafes' and 'Internet Providers'. Your local library offers a similar facility and has staff to help you find the information that you need.

It should always be remembered, however, that the internet is unregulated and anyone is free to set up a website and add information to it. Many websites offer impartial advice and information that has been compiled and checked by qualified medical professionals. Some, on the other hand, are run by commercial organisations with the purpose of promoting their own products. Others still are run by pressure groups, some of which will provide carefully assessed and accurate information whereas others may be suggesting medications or treatments that are not supported by the medical and scientific community.

Unless you know the address of the website you want to visit – for example, www.familydoctor.co.uk – you may find the following guidelines useful when searching the internet for information.

### Search engines and other searchable sites

Google (www.google.co.uk) is the most popular search engine used in the UK, followed by Yahoo! (http://uk.yahoo.com) and MSN (www.msn.co.uk). Also popular are the search engines provided by Internet Service Providers such as Tiscali and other sites such as the BBC site (www.bbc.co.uk).

In addition to the search engines that index the whole web, there are also medical sites with search facilities, which act almost like mini-search engines, but cover only medical topics or even a particular area of medicine. Again, it is wise to look at who is responsible for compiling the information offered to ensure that it is impartial and medically accurate. The NHS Direct site (www.nhsdirect.nhs.uk) is an example of a searchable medical site.

Links to many British medical charities can be found at the Association of Medical Research Charities' website (www.amrc.org.uk) and at Charity Choice (www.charitychoice.co.uk).

### Search phrases

Be specific when entering a search phrase. Searching for information on 'cancer' will return results for many different types of cancer as well as on cancer in general. You may even find sites offering astrological information. More useful results will be returned by using search phrases such as 'lung cancer' and 'treatments for lung cancer'. Both Google and Yahoo! offer an advanced search option that includes the ability to search for the exact phrase; enclosing the search phrase in quotes, that is, 'treatments for lung cancer', will have the same effect. Limiting a search to an exact phrase reduces the number of results returned but it is best to refine a search to an exact match only if you are not getting useful results with a normal search. Adding 'UK' to your search term will bring up mainly British sites, so a good phrase might be 'lung cancer' UK (don't include UK within the quotes).

Always remember the internet is international and unregulated. It holds a wealth of valuable information but individual sites may be biased, out of date or just plain wrong. Family Doctor Publications accepts no responsibility for the content of links published in this series.

# Index

acupuncture **91–2**
 – British Acupuncture
    Council **114**
adalimumab (Humira) **27–8,
    81–2**
adhesive capsulitis (frozen
    shoulder) **54–6**
adrenal glands, effect of
    steroids **79, 80**
aerobic exercise **103**
African–Caribbean origins,
    SLE **41**
alcohol consumption **34**
Alexander technique **92–3**
 – Society of Teachers of the
    Alexander Technique
    **121–2**
allopurinol **33–4**
anaemia **11, 23, 26**
analgesics **72**
 – guidelines for use **73**
 – use in osteoarthritis **19, 20**
ankles, stretching exercises
    **102**

ankylosing spondylitis **36–7,
    52**
 – National Ankylosing
    Spondylitis Association **118**
anti-inflammatory drugs *see*
    non-steroidal anti-
    inflammatory drugs
antidepressant drugs **83**
anxiety **8**
appetite loss **23**
Arava (leflunomide) **27, 81**
Arcoxia (etoricoxib) **74**
arthralgia **9**
arthritis
 – in children **39**
 – what it is **1**
 – *see also* ankylosing
    spondylitis; osteoarthritis;
    psoriatic arthritis; reactive
    arthritis; rheumatoid
    arthritis
Arthritis Care **112–13**
Arthritis and Musculoskeletal
    Alliance (ARMA) **112**

Arthritis Research Campaign
     41, 113
arthroplasty (joint replacement)
     20, 86–7, 88
arthroscopy 84, 85
artificial joints 20, 86–7, 88
aspirin 72, 77
   – avoidance in gout 34
Assist UK 113
Association of Medical
     Research Charities 124
asthma, caution with NSAIDs
     77
athrodesis 86, 87
autoimmune connective
     tissue diseases 22
azathioprine 27, 81

back, stretching exercises
     99–100
back pain 48–9
   – ankylosing spondylitis
     36–7
   – osteoporosis 52–3
   – spondylosis 51–2
BackCare 114
Benefits Enquiry Line 114
big toe, gout 31
biologics (biological agents)
     27–8
blood pressure, possible
     effect of steroids 78
blood tests 10–12
   – in diagnosis of gout 32
   – in diagnosis of
     rheumatoid arthritis 26
   – in DMARD therapy 28
blue card, steroid therapy
     79
body mass index (BMI) 108

Bodytalkonline 122
bones
   – skeleton 2
   – thinning of (osteoporosis)
     52–3
bony overgrowth
     (osteophytes) 14, 16,
     17
breathlessness 24
British Acupuncture Council
     114
British Association of
     Occupational Therapists
     115
British Homeopathic
     Association 115
bursas 4, 5, 53

caffeine intake 46
calcium, loss from bones 53
calcium pyrophosphate 32
capitate bone 60
capsule of joints 3–4
Care directions 122
carpal bones 60
carpal tunnel syndrome 61,
     64–5, 81
cartilage 3, 4
   – changes in osteoarthritis
     16, 17
   – changes in rheumatoid
     arthritis 22, 23
   – of knee joint (meniscus)
     68
case histories
   – osteoarthritis 5–6
   – rheumatoid arthritis 6–7
celecoxib (Celebrex) 74
chairs 104
Charity Choice 123

Chartered Society of Physiotherapy 116
children, arthritis 39
Children's Chronic Arthritis Association (CCAA) 115
chiropractic 92, 93
chondroitin sulphate 89, 91
clavicle (collar bone) 2
clicking fingers 66–7
Clinical Knowledge Summaries 116
co-dydramol 72
co-proxamol 72
cod liver oil 91
codeine 72
colchicine 32
collateral ligaments, knee joint 68
complementary medicine 87, 89, 93
 – acupuncture 91–2
 – fish oils 91
 – glucosamine and chondroitin sulphate 89, 91
 – guidelines 90
 – homoeopathy 92
 – osteopathy, chiropractic and Alexander technique 92–3
computer use, avoidance of RSI 62–3
connective tissue diseases 41–2
constipation, as side effect of medication 72
Contact a Family 116
cool weather, effect on symptoms 105
copper bracelets 89

COX-2 inhibitors 74–6
creaking joints (crepitus) 18
Crossroads Association 117
cruciate ligaments 68

de Quervain's tenosynovitis (thumb tendinitis) 65–6
degeneration 15
depression 8, 43, 46
dermatomyositis 42
diabetes, as side effect of medication 78
diagnosis 14
 – of gout 32, 33
 – of osteoarthritis 18–19
 – of PMR 43
 – of rheumatoid arthritis 26
diarrhoea, as side effect of medication 32
diclofenac 72
diet 106–7
 – avoidance of gout 34
dihydrocodeine 72
Disabled Living Foundation 103, 117
discs, prolapsed (slipped) 49–50
disease-modifying anti-rheumatoid drugs (DMARDs) 27–8, 81–2
dislocations, in hypermobility 47
dizziness 18
doctors, what they will do
 – blood tests 10–12
 – history taking 9–10
 – physical examination 10
 – X-rays 12–14
'double-jointedness' 47

'dowager's hump' 53
drowsiness, as side effect of medication 72
drug treatments 71, 93
 – analgesics 72, 73
 – antidepressant drugs 83
 – DMARDs 81–2
 – NSAIDs 72, 74–6, 77
 – steroids 76, 78–81

elbow pain 58–9
elbows, stretching exercises 97
Enbrel (etanercept) 27–8, 81–2
endorphins 91
erosions 13, 22, 23
essential fatty acids 91
ESR (erythrocyte sedimentation rate) 11–12, 26
 – in PMR 43
etanercept (Enbrel) 27–8, 81–2
etoricoxib (Arcoxia) 74
evening primrose oil 91
examination by doctor 10
exclusion diets 106
exercise 53, 71, 83, 94–5, 109, 111
 – aerobic 103
 – in ankylosing spondylitis 37
 – in fibromyalgia 46
 – for frozen shoulder 55–6
 – in hypermobility 47
 – in osteoarthritis 6, 19
 – for shoulder tendinitis 56
 – strengthening 102
 – stretching 95–102
exercise bicycles 103

extensor muscle attachment, tennis elbow 59
eye problems
 – in ankylosing spondylitis 37
 – in juvenile idiopathic arthritis 39
 – in rheumatoid arthritis 24

family history 9, 107
 – of ankylosing spondylitis 36
 – of osteoarthritis 15
feet, stretching exercises 102
femur (thigh bone) 2
fever 23
fibromyalgia 45–6
 – Fibromyalgia Association UK 117
fibula 2
fingers, tender lumps 18
fish oils 91
flares of rheumatoid arthritis 24, 29
flu, as cause of pain 9
fluid, removal from joints 18, 32, 33
fluid intake, prevention of gout 34
fluid retention, carpal tunnel syndrome 61
food allergies 106
foot, anatomy 70
frozen shoulder (adhesive capsulitis) 54–6
full blood count 10–11, 26
fusion of joints 86, 87

gel preparations, NSAIDs 77

gender differences
– in ankylosing spondylitis 36
– in fibromyalgia 45
– in gout 30
– in SLE 41
General Osteopathic Council 118
glucosamine 89, 91
gold salts 27, 81
golfer's elbow 58
gout 12
– diagnosis 32, 33
– diet 106
– prevention 33–5
– symptoms 31
– treatment 32, 76
– what happens 30–1
– who gets it 30

haemoglobin level 11
hair, thinning of 42
hamate bone 60
hands
– anatomy 60
– stretching exercises 98
– tender lumps 18
headaches 18, 51
Healthtalkonline 122
heart attacks 54
– risk from COX-2 inhibitors 74–5
heat, soothing effect 105, 110
heel cups 69
heel pain (plantar fasciitis) 37, 67–70
height, loss of 52, 53
help, where to find it
– searching the internet 122–4

– useful addresses 112–21
– websites 121–2
herbal remedies 89
hip replacement 87, 88
hips
– osteoarthritis 5–6
– stretching exercises 100–1
history taking 9–10
HLA-B27 37
homoeopathy 92
– British Homeopathic Association 115
hospital clinics, staff 25
hospital referral 14
hot packs 110
humerus 2
Humira (adalimumab) 27–8, 81–2
hydrotherapy 83–4
hydroxychloroquine 27, 81–2
hypermobility 47–8
Hypermobility Syndrome Association 118

ibuprofen 72, 77
ice packs 110
indigestion, as side effect of medication 74, 75, 77
infections
– as cause of arthritis 9, 37–8
– increased susceptibility 79
inflammation
– ESR as marker 11–12
– in rheumatoid arthritis 22, 23, 24
inflammatory arthritis 21, 36
– ankylosing spondylitis 36–7
– psoriatic arthritis 38–9

– reactive arthritis (Reiter's syndrome) 37–8
– see also rheumatoid arthritis
inflammatory bowel disease 9, 38
infliximab (Remicade) 27, 81–2
infrapatellar bursa 5
inheritance of arthritis 9, 107
injections into joints 18, 81, 82
injuries, history of 9, 15, 16
investigations
– blood tests 10–12
– in rheumatoid arthritis 26
– X-rays 12–14

joint replacement surgery 20, 86–7, 88
joint space, reduced 13
joints
– changes in gout 30–1
– changes in osteoarthritis 16, 17
– changes in rheumatoid arthritis 22–3
– how they work 3–4
– steroid injections 81, 82
juvenile idiopathic arthritis 39

keyboard use, avoidance of RSI 62–3
'keyhole' surgery (arthroscopy) 84, 85
kidneys, in gout 31
kitchen, protecting your joints 104
knee joints
– anatomy 68
– arthroscopy 85
– bursas 5
– looking after them 69
– stretching exercises 101
knee pain 67
knee replacement 87, 88

leflunomide (Arava) 27, 81
leg pain, sciatica 49–50
lifestyle changes, fibromyalgia 46
lifting, as trigger for elbow pain 58
ligament surgery 85
ligaments 3, 4
– of knee joint 68
locomotor system 1
lumbago (back pain) 48–9
lumbar spine, stretching exercises 99–100
lumiracoxib (Prexige) 74
lunate bone 60
lungs, problems in rheumatoid arthritis 24

MabThera (rituximab) 27, 81–2
massage 110
mechanical back pain 48
median nerve, carpal tunnel syndrome 61, 64–5
meniscus (cartilage) of knee joint 68
metacarpals 60
methotrexate 27, 81–2
miscarriages 42
mobilise 118
morning stiffness
– in ankylosing spondylitis 37

morning stiffness (contd)
- in fibromyalgia 46
- in PMR 43
- in rheumatoid arthritis 23, 24
multidisciplinary treatment 71
muscle-strengthening exercises 102
muscle weakness, polymyositis 42

nails, changes in psoriatic arthritis 38
naproxen 72
National Ankylosing Spondylitis Association (NASS) 118–19
National Institute for Health and Clinical Excellence (NICE) 91, 119
National Osteoporosis Society 119
National Rheumatoid Arthritis Society 120
neck arthritis, symptoms 18
neck exercises 94, 95–6
neck pain 51
nerve irritation, prolapsed (slipped) discs 49, 50
nerve root irritation, symptoms 18
neuralgia, use of antidepressant drugs 83
NHS choices 120
NHS Direct 120
NHS Smoking Helpline 120
Night-time pain 73
nodules, in rheumatoid arthritis 24
non-specific back pain 48

non-steroidal anti-inflammatory drugs (NSAIDs) 72, 76
- COX-2 inhibitors 74–6
- effects on stomach 74, 75
- guidelines for use 77
- use in gout 32
- use in rheumatoid arthritis 27
numbness 18
- in hand 64
nurse specialists 25

obesity 108, 109
occupational therapists 7, 25, 103, 105
- British Association of Occupational Therapists 114
orthopaedic surgeons 14, 25
osteoarthritis 109
- case history 5–6
- changes in joints 16, 17
- diagnosis 18–19
- family history 15
- how common it is 15
- outlook 19–20
- reduced joint space 13
- symptoms 16, 18
- treatment 19, 76
- which joints are affected 16
osteopathy 92, 93
- General Osteopathic Council 117
osteophytes 14, 16, 17
osteoporosis 52–3
- National Osteoporosis Society 119

osteoporosis, as side effect of medication 79
osteotomy 85, 86
outlook
– in osteoarthritis 19–20
– in rheumatoid arthritis 28–9
overuse syndrome (repetitive strain injury, RSI) 59–61, 109
– self-help tips 62–3
overweight 108, 109

pain 8, 9
– in ankylosing spondylitis 37
– around elbow 58–9
– in gout 31
– in hand 64
– in knees 67
– neck pain 51
– in osteoarthritis 18
– sciatica 49
– see also back pain; shoulder pain
pain control 107, 109, 110
pain-killers (analgesics) 72
– guidelines for use 73
– use in osteoarthritis 19, 20
paracetamol 72, 73
– use with NSAIDs 77
patella (kneecap) 2, 68
patellar ligament 5, 68
Patient UK 122
Patients' Association 120–1
pelvis, joints 3
penicillamine 27, 81
physical examination 10
physiotherapy 7, 25, 71, 83, 105

– Chartered Society of Physiotherapy 115
– value in ankylosing spondylitis 37
pins and needles 18, 49
pitting of nails 38
plantar fasciitis 67–70
podiatrists 25
polymyalgia rheumatica (PMR) 42–3, 78
polymyositis 42
posture 109
– Alexander technique 92–3
– avoidance of RSI 63
– as cause of neck pain 51
prepatellar bursa 5
Prexige (lumiracoxib) 74
prolapsed discs 49–50
prostaglandins 74
protecting your joints 103–5
pseudogout 32
psoriasis 9
psoriatic arthritis 38–9
purines 30
– which foods contain them 34

Quit (Smoking Quitlines) 121

RADAR 121
radius 2
rashes 24
– in SLE 42
reactive arthritis (Reiter's syndrome) 9, 37–8
realignment of bones (osteotomy) 85, 86
red blood cells 11

relapses, rheumatoid arthritis
    **24**, **29**
relaxation **46**
Remicade (infliximab) **27**,
    **81–2**
remissions, rheumatoid
    arthritis **24**
repetitive strain injury (RSI,
    overuse syndrome)
    **59–61**, **109**
– self-help tips **62–3**
rest **94**
rheumatism **1**
rheumatoid arthritis
– anaemia **11**
– carpal tunnel syndrome
    **61**
– case history **6–7**
– changes in joints **22–3**
– diagnosis **26**
– erosions **13**
– National Rheumatoid
    Arthritis Society **119**
– outlook **28–9**
– symptoms **23–4**
– treatment **26–8**, **76**
    – steroid injections **81**
    – synovectomy **84**
– what it is **21**
– which joints are affected
    **23**
rheumatoid disease **21**
rheumatoid factor **12**, **26**
rheumatoid nodules **24**
rheumatologists **14**, **25**
ribs **2**
rituximab (MabThera) **27**,
    **81–2**
ruptured (slipped) discs **49–50**

sacroiliac joints
– in ankylosing spondylitis
    **36**
– in psoriatic arthritis **39**
scaphoid bone **60**
scapula (shoulder blade) **2**
sciatica **49–50**
shingles **54**
shoes **104**
shopping bags **57–8**
shoulder joints
– anatomy **57**
– stretching exercises **96–7**
shoulder pain **54**
– frozen shoulder **54–6**
– tendinitis **56–8**
side effects of medication
– analgesics **72**
– aspirin **72**
– colchicine **32**
– local steroid injections **81**
– NSAIDs **74**, **75**, **77**
– steroids **78–9**
simple analgesics **72**
skeleton **2**
skin, effects of steroids **79**,
    **81**
skull **2**
– joints **3**
SLE *see* systemic lupus
    erythematosus
sleep disturbance
– in fibromyalgia **45**, **46**
– in frozen shoulder **54**
'slipped discs' **49–50**
smoking
– NHS Smoking Helpline
    **120**
– Quit (Smoking Quitlines)
    **121**

social workers **25**
Society of Teachers of the
   Alexander Technique
   (STAT) **121–2**
soft-tissue rheumatism **53–4**
specialist nurses **25**
specialist referral **14**
spine
 – arthritis of **51–2**
 – bony overgrowth
   (osteophytes) **14**
 – stretching exercises
   **99–100**
spondyloarthritis **37–9**
spondylosis **51–2**
sports injuries **54**
spurs, plantar fasciitis **68, 70**
squat exercises **94**
sternum (breast bone) **2**
steroid injections **18, 53, 78,
   81, 82**
 – for carpal tunnel
   syndrome **65**
 – for elbow pain **58**
 – for frozen shoulder **55**
 – for plantar fasciitis **69**
 – for shoulder tendinitis **56**
 – for thumb tendinitis
   **65–6**
 – for trigger finger **67**
steroids **28, 76**
 – guidelines for long-term
   use **79**
 – possible side effects **78–9**
 – stopping treatment **80, 90**
 – use in connective tissue
   disorders **42**
 – use in PMR **43**
 – ways in which they can
   be taken **78**

stiffness **8**
 – in ankylosing spondylitis
   **37**
 – in fibromyalgia **46**
 – in frozen shoulder **55**
 – in osteoarthritis **18**
 – in PMR **43**
 – in rheumatoid arthritis
   **23, 24**
stomach, effects of NSAIDs
   **74, 75, 77**
strengthening exercises **102**
stress
 – as trigger for fibromyalgia
   **45**
 – as trigger for flares **29**
stretching exercises **95–102**
strokes, risk from COX-2
   inhibitors **74–5**
sulfasalazine **27, 81**
suprapatellar bursa **5**
surgery **84–7, 88**
 – in osteoarthritis **20**
swelling **8**
 – in rheumatoid arthritis **23**
swimming **103**
symptom diaries **90**
symptoms **8–9**
 – of ankylosing spondylitis
   **37**
 – of carpal tunnel
   syndrome **64**
 – describing them **9–10**
 – effect of weather **105**
 – of fibromyalgia **45–6**
 – of frozen shoulder **54–5**
 – of gout **31**
 – of osteoarthritis **16, 18**
 – of PMR **43**
 – of psoriatic arthritis **38–9**

symptoms (contd)
- of rheumatoid arthritis 23–4
- of SLE 42
synovectomy 84
synovial fluid 4
synovial joints 3–4
synovium 3, 4, 17
- changes in rheumatoid arthritis 22, 23
systemic lupus erythematosus (SLE, lupus) 41–2, 78

tendinitis
- of shoulder 56–8
- of thumb 65–6
tendon sheaths 4, 6
tendon surgery 85
tendons 53
tennis elbow 58–9, 81
TENS (transcutaneous electrical nerve stimulation) 110
tension headaches 51
tests see investigations
thigh muscles, exercises 69
thoracic spine, stretching exercises 99
thumb tendinitis 65–6
thyroid gland underactivity 61
tibia 2
tingling, in hand 64
tiredness 45
tophi 31
trapezium bone 60
trapezius muscle 54
trapezoid bone 60
treatment 93
- of carpal tunnel syndrome 65

- complementary medicine 87, 89–93
- of frozen shoulder 55
- of gout 32
- hydrotherapy 83–4
- multidisciplinary approach 71
- of osteoarthritis 19
- of overuse syndrome 60–1
- physiotherapy 83
- of PMR 43
- of prolapsed (slipped) discs 49
- of rheumatoid arthritis 26–8
- of shoulder tendinitis 56
- surgery 84–7
- of SLE 42
- of thumb tendinitis 65–6
- see also drug treatments
trigger finger 66–7
triquetrum bone 60

ulcerative colitis 9, 38
ulcers 24
- as side effect of medication 74, 75, 77, 79
ulna 2
upper limb syndrome (RSI) 59–61, 109
- self-help tips 62–3
uric acid
- blood levels 12, 32
- effect of allopurinol 33
- in gout 30
uric acid crystals 32, 33
urine tests, in DMARD therapy 28

vasculitis 24
vertebrae 2
 – collapse of 52, 53
vitamin A 91
vitamin D 91

walking sticks 104–5
wear and tear 15
weather, effect on symptoms
     105
weight 34
 – what you should weigh
     108
weight-bearing exercise 95
weight gain, as side effect of
     medication 78
weight loss 23, 43

weight reduction 83
 – benefits to knees 69
 – value in osteoarthritis 19
 – value in plantar fasciitis
     68, 69
weights, strengthening
     exercises 102
white blood cells 11
wrist splints 65
wrists
 – anatomy 60
 – anatomy of carpal tunnel
     64
 – stretching exercises 98

X-rays 12–14, 26, 51

# Your pages

We have included the following pages because they may help you manage your illness or condition and its treatment.

Before an appointment with a health professional, it can be useful to write down a short list of questions of things that you do not understand, so that you can make sure that you do not forget anything.

Some of the sections may not be relevant to your circumstances.

We are always pleased to receive constructive criticism or suggestions about how to improve the books. You can contact us at:

Email:   familydoctor@btinternet.com
Letter:  Family Doctor Publications
         PO Box 4664
         Poole
         BH15 1NN

*Thank you*

## Health-care contact details

Name:

Job title:

Place of work:


Tel:


Name:

Job title:

Place of work:


Tel:


Name:

Job title:

Place of work:


Tel:


Name:

Job title:

Place of work:


Tel:

## Significant past health events – illnesses/operations/investigations/treatments

| Event | Month | Year | Age (at time) |
|-------|-------|------|---------------|
|       |       |      |               |
|       |       |      |               |
|       |       |      |               |
|       |       |      |               |
|       |       |      |               |
|       |       |      |               |
|       |       |      |               |
|       |       |      |               |
|       |       |      |               |
|       |       |      |               |
|       |       |      |               |
|       |       |      |               |
|       |       |      |               |
|       |       |      |               |
|       |       |      |               |
|       |       |      |               |
|       |       |      |               |
|       |       |      |               |
|       |       |      |               |
|       |       |      |               |

## Appointments for health care

Name:

Place:

Date:

Time:

Tel:


Name:

Place:

Date:

Time:

Tel:


Name:

Place:

Date:

Time:

Tel:


Name:

Place:

Date:

Time:

Tel:

## Appointments for health care

Name:

Place:

Date:

Time:

Tel:

Name:

Place:

Date:

Time:

Tel:

Name:

Place:

Date:

Time:

Tel:

Name:

Place:

Date:

Time:

Tel:

**Current medication(s) prescribed by your doctor**

Medicine name:

Purpose:

Frequency & dose:

Start date:

End date:

Medicine name:

Purpose:

Frequency & dose:

Start date:

End date:

Medicine name:

Purpose:

Frequency & dose:

Start date:

End date:

Medicine name:

Purpose:

Frequency & dose:

Start date:

End date:

## Other medicines/supplements you are taking, not prescribed by your doctor

Medicine/treatment:

Purpose:

Frequency & dose:

Start date:

End date:

Medicine/treatment:

Purpose:

Frequency & dose:

Start date:

End date:

Medicine/treatment:

Purpose:

Frequency & dose:

Start date:

End date:

Medicine/treatment:

Purpose:

Frequency & dose:

Start date:

End date:

## Questions to ask at appointments

(Note: do bear in mind that doctors work under great time pressure, so long lists may not be helpful for either of you)

## Questions to ask at appointments
(Note: do bear in mind that doctors work under great time pressure, so long lists may not be helpful for either of you)

**Notes**